# eating
## in
## the
# raw

# eating
# in
# the

# raw

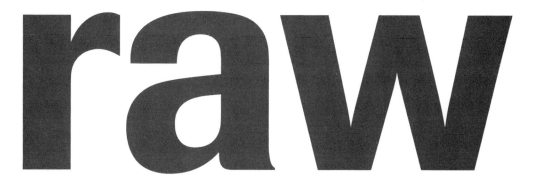

a beginner's guide
to getting slimmer,
feeling healthier,
and
living longer
the raw-food way

## carol alt

WITH DAVID ROTH

**foreword by nicholas j. gonzalez, m.d.**

clarkson potter/publishers
new york

Published by Clarkson Potter/Publishers, New York, New York.
Member of the Crown Publishing Group, a division of Random House, Inc.
www.randomhouse.com

CLARKSON N. POTTER is a trademark and POTTER and colophon are registered trademarks of Random House, Inc.

Printed in the United States of America

Design by Jane Treuhaft

Library of Congress Cataloging-in-Publication Data
Alt, Carol, 1960–
    Eating in the raw : a beginner's guide to getting slimmer, feeling healthier, and living longer the raw-food way / Carol Alt, with David Roth
    1. Weight loss.   2. Reducing diets.   3. Raw food diet.   4. Health.
I. Roth, David, 1955–   II. Title.
    RM237.5.A465   2004
    613.2'5—dc22      2004010506

ISBN 1-4000-5284-x

10  9  8  7  6  5  4  3

First Edition

# a brief note before we begin

This is a chronicle of my experience with raw foods. It is not intended as a medical manual, or as a substitute for informed medical advice. As with any diet or lifestyle change, you should consult with your own doctor before starting. While this book emphasizes the benefits of eating uncooked foods, raw meat, fish, dairy, and eggs, these ingredients (especially from an unreliable source) can contain bacteria that may cause serious illness or even death. People who are pregnant or have suppressed immune systems are especially vulnerable. Please consult a medical resource if you are unsure about the health risks of any foods.

–Carol Alt

# contents

# foreword
## nicholas j. gonzalez, m.d.

This book tells the story of raw food—why it is beneficial and how to begin the raw-food journey. Before that journey begins, however, I'd like to share some insights into the science *behind* raw food, explaining just why eating raw affects the body the way it does. And it all has to do with enzymes.

Enzymes are indeed the spark of life. Without them, no flower could bloom, no human could think, no cell could live; in fact, life as we know it would not be possible. Despite such importance, most of us might not care much about enzymes, or even know what they are. We probably are all familiar with DNA, the basic genetic material of cells, the substance of our genes, which in the media, on television, and at scientific conferences gets all the publicity and grabs the spotlight. We hear on a near weekly basis about gene technology, the Genome Project to map our human chromosomes, gene therapy to treat all manner of degenerative and inherited disease. But we don't hear much about enzymes; though I've seen literally dozens of stories in the popular press discussing the miracles of our genes, I don't recall, other than articles written about my work, any articles highlighting enzymes, what they do, their role in health, and importantly, their potential as a treatment for human disease. There are, to my knowledge, no noteworthy conferences devoted to these molecules, no PowerPoint press releases extolling their significance, no TV specials to glamorize, or mystify.

They deserve more attention, certainly. But what, actually, are these molecules, these sparks of life, as I call them? Enzymes are first, and foremost, *proteins*. We all have some idea of what a protein is: it's the material that makes up our muscle; it's the shaft of our hair, the stuff of our nails, the gel in Knox gelatin we take to strengthen those nails.

To a biochemist, proteins are interesting molecules, consisting, as they all do, of complex arrays of amino acids, their basic bricks or building blocks. There are some twenty-four or so amino acids used by us humans, including eight *essen-*

*tial* amino acids, so called because we cannot make them in our cells, and they must be provided like a vitamin or mineral in the diet. The other sixteen we can manufacture from molecules such as glucose or even from other amino acids.

Enzymes are protein *catalysts,* that is, a molecule that allows a chemical reaction to occur efficiently, with a minimal amount of energy needed to get the process, whatever it may be, going. Enzymes essentially allow things to happen easily. For example, there are reactions in all our cells that without catalysts would require thousands of degrees of temperature, and thousands of years to come to completion, but with these molecules present, can happen within milliseconds at our comfortable temperature of 98.6 degrees. You can see, then, why without enzymes, there would be no life at all. A thousand degrees of heat would vaporize any cell, very very quickly.

Enzymes do many things, both within our cells and without. They help produce chemical energy to fuel our cells and their many varied activities. Our immune cells, our neurotrophils and lymphocytes, use enzymes to attack and kill bacteria, viruses, and fungi, as well as dangerous cancer cells that some scientists believe form every day in all of us. In the nucleus, another set of these unusual proteins allow DNA to repair itself from the ravages of free radicals and other toxic assaults, and in fact, without certain enzymes our genetic material could not duplicate itself as needed for cell division. That's a pretty important assignment, when you consider that, for example, the lining of the intestinal tract replaces itself every five days, and without these nuclear enzymes such efficient turnover would be impossible. So, though DNA gets the headlines, without enzymes it can do nothing.

And outside the cells, in the stomach and small intestine, digestive enzymes such as pepsin and sucrase released by the gut lining help break down proteins and carbohydrates to jump start the digestive process. And importantly, at the back of the upper abdomen sits the pancreas, a most powerful gland that produces insulin, to regulate sugar metabolism and dozens of enzymes without which efficient digestion would be impossible.

Not surprisingly, enzymes, as busy as they are, wear out and need to be replaced. Our bodies—our tissues and cells—have the ability to make the enzymes we need from the basic amino acids provided by food, or available through cellular recycling. But this process, as useful as it is, has its drawbacks;

enzymes are complicated molecules, sometimes consisting of thousands of amino acids, that must be aligned in a very precise order—one out of line, and the enzyme will most likely not be able to carry out its assigned responsibility. It's a difficult undertaking to make so many of these molecules, an effort that requires energy enzymes. Certainly, we can make the enzymes we need, but it would make sense if we didn't have to expend time, and metabolic effort, and energy creating and replacing worn out and lost proteins. Think of it, in every second there are thousands of reactions going on in every cell, each usually involving a series of steps that require at every point a different enzyme—it's a major manufacturing job to keep those catalysts in adequate supply.

It would be helpful, from a thermodynamic perspective, if we could get our enzymes preformed, premade, ready to go to work, without always having to start from scratch. It would save time, effort, and energy.

There is a way, of course, and that way is from our food. But, as we shall see, only from *raw food.* Enzymes are indeed wonderful molecules, extraordinarily complex in their design and in their behavior, but like most proteins, they are very sensitive to heat. At around 106–107 degrees F., enzymes begin deteriorating, and above 116 degrees, most *denature*—that is, they become completely inactive, unable to do anything useful in the cell. That's why fevers above 107 degrees F. are generally deadly, because at that point our enzymes start self-destructing, throughout all our tissues.

When we cook food, we change it in many ways; scientists have known for years that heat inactivates certain vitamins such as folic acid and vitamin C, and at sustained, high temperatures, certain minerals, such as calcium, become less readily absorbed. All this is true—when you cook food, you change certain vitamins for the worse, and you make certain minerals less biologically accessible, but what even nutritional scientists in general ignore is that when you cook food, you *very quickly destroy all its enzymes.* Keep in mind that food, whether it be of plant or animal origin, a fruit, vegetable, nut, seed, grain product, egg, piece of fish, or cut of meat—are themselves made up of cells, all loaded with their own cast of enzymes. Depending on the type of food, these food enzymes, as some have called them, can stay active for prolonged periods of time, particularly if refrigerated, since cold temperatures slow down their deterioration. Those in nuts and seeds, protected by a tough outer coat, seem able to last eternally, and even wheat grains buried with the pharaohs thousands of years ago can germinate under the right conditions—a process that requires active enzymes. But as soon as you cook them, the enzymes are dead, forever.

So, when you cook food, be it fruit, vegetable, nut, seed, grain, egg, dairy, fish, poultry, meat—all the enzymes are gone, very quickly. The body can use its own enzymes in the digestive tract to break these denatured proteins down into the component amino acids, absorb them as such, then put them back together into brand new enzymes—a process that is, again, time and energy consuming, and amounts to basically reinventing a very complicated wheel.

Edward Howell, the underappreciated American physician and scientist, first proposed during the 1920s and 1930s that raw food contains living, vital enzymes in their active form—enzymes that can be absorbed, much like a vita-min or mineral, from the digestive tract, and be used by our cells to replenish our own stock of worn or defective catalysts. This was a controversial claim that few scientists in Howell's day, and few today, would accept. First, the usual objection raised then and now is that enzymes are themselves proteins, and like any ingested protein, will be broken down in the gut into the constitutive amino acids during the digestive process. However, in meticulously performed studies, Howell showed over and over again that in humans and in animals, these com-plicated molecules largely survive digestion, are absorbed, and seem to be reused. More recently, the research team of Drs. Liebow and Rothman have, over a twenty-five-year period, documented again that certain pancreatic enzymes, as complicated as they are, are taken up in the gut, intact and active.

Howell actually came to these conclusions out of his experiences trying to find a solution for his own declining health. Apparently, in his twenties he became quite ill, to the point he thought he would be unable to continue his medical career. From what I've read, his symptoms seem consistent with what we might today call Chronic Fatigue Syndrome, persistent exhaustion and malaise so severe he was virtually non-functional. He consulted a variety of doctors, both orthodox and unconventional, with no results, until he finally put himself on a complete raw-foods diet. I want to emphasize that the eating plan Howell himself followed was not vegetarian, but included raw eggs, raw dairy products, even raw meat, along with juices, raw fruits, raw vegetables, and sprouted raw nuts, seeds, and grains. This eating approach was the only therapy that made any difference in his health, and, research scientist that he was, he carefully studied the diet that had brought him back to exuberant well-being. To him, it wasn't the vitamins and minerals that made the difference, though he knew some of these might be affected by cooking—when he had previously taken vitamin or mineral concentrates, he had felt no better. What he thought ultimately cured him were the enzymes in the raw food, these protein catalysts that he now believed must be absorbed in a usable and potent form.

With his health renewed, Howell began to apply what he had learned and continued to do so with thousands of patients over the span of a fifty-year career. And over and over, he reported what he found in himself, that when all else failed, raw food could frequently help. In his two published books, Howell discusses his experiences and cites hundreds of scientific studies of both laboratory animals and humans to support his contention that raw is best.

Another scientist who made a strong case for the value of raw over cooked food was the University of Southern California physician Francis Pottenger, a most interesting character. Trained in the early twentieth century as an expert in tuberculosis, a rampant disease at the time, Pottenger's interests were wide-ranging: he wrote a text on neurophysiology, for example, that is still a classic. For our purposes, of greatest import are the series of cat studies he completed during the 1930s. These were simple experiments, to be sure; repeatedly, he would separate two groups of cats, feed one a completely raw meat, raw milk diet, and feed the other nothing but cooked meat and pasteurized milk. He would follow the cats through multiple generations, feeding the offspring in the same way as the parents, so the kittens of raw-food cats got nothing but raw, and those with parents eating cooked food, got the cooked. Simple enough, indeed. But the results were extraordinary: in the raw-foods group, the cats remained, through generation after generation, healthy and happy, with normal bone structure, healthy fur, and a resistance to allergies, arthritis, eye problems, and other degenerative diseases. They were happy cats who lived in peace with each other in their cat world. The cooked-food cats, after only one or two generations, suffered an epidemic of abnormalities in the bones, chronic skin problems, allergies, arthritis, and a host of degenerative illnesses. These animals also exhibited all manner of anti-social behavior to the point that their cat society began to break down. By the third generation, the animals were so deteriorated they could not even reproduce and the line came to an end. Each time Pottenger repeated the experiments, the results were the same: the raw-food animals stayed wonderfully healthy, generation after generation, the cooked-food animals suffered and eventually died out.

These were extraordinary results, but largely ignored by the mainstream medical world. But, like Howell, Pottenger made a clear and persuasive case that though we humans take cooked food for granted, raw and cooked are not the same. And the difference must be the enzymes.

What Howell claimed and what Pottenger observed really shouldn't be that surprising. I have long found it interesting that of all the millions upon millions of animal species that have existed since life began, we are the only one that cooks its food. No other species has done that, not fruit flies, not gorillas, not dinosaurs; in nature, it's all raw. Of course, our dog and cat pets eat cooked food, but that's only because they hang around us, and like us, they also now suffer an epidemic of degenerative diseases, including cancer. But certainly, cooking, which we all take for granted, is an extraordinary change to have made in something so vital as our food, and a change that scientists and anthropologists generally ignore despite the work of men like Howell and Pottenger.

There is another name, another man, that deserves mentioning, Dr. John Beard, the Scotsman who at the turn of the last century first suggested that the pancreatic proteolytic enzyme trypsin represents the body's main defense against cancer, and would be useful as a cancer treatment. Even then, scientists recognized that trypsin was one of the main digestive enzymes, but prior to Beard it was thought to have no other function. Beard's thesis, revolutionary and controversial at the time, remains revolutionary and controversial today, a hundred years later. But his life's work with enzymes has been the impetus of my own research career, since I first heard his name while a medical student at Cornell.

In our office today, we continue in the traditions of Howell, Pottenger, and Beard, and use enzymes against cancer and other degenerative diseases. We have already completed our first clinical trial, in which we treated patients with advanced pancreatic cancer with large doses of proteolytic enzymes. Fortunately, the results were substantial enough to warrant a National Cancer Institute–National Center for Complementary and Alternative Medicine grant to study our approach in a large-scale clinical effort. So we are making progress—the work of scientists such as Beard is finally being properly tested, and hopefully, someday, deservedly recognized.

I was pleased when I learned that my friend Carol Alt intended to write a book about raw foods, and how a raw-foods approach made such a difference in her own health. Her personal story is inspiring, and I always think it useful when ideas that have remained largely hidden are brought into the open for discussion and review. I admire Carol, as busy as she is, for taking the time to share, in her own way, what raw foods and enzymes have done for her. I wish her well with her effort, and continued good health.

# introduction

For a quarter century, I've been scrutinized by the cameras of some of the world's greatest photographers and by the public eye. Now, people who have known me for many years come up to me and tell me that they can't believe the way I look. ✳ Makeup artists, many of them too young to know any of my early work, are usually surprised to find out how old I am and, when they do find out, routinely tell me that I don't look anywhere near my age. They seem to think that in my forties I should appear a lot older than I do. Of course I'm flattered, but mostly I'm grateful. ✳ The first question I'm asked is, "What's your secret?" I have to tell them first of all that I try to be careful about what I put on my skin, so I partnered with QVC on a line of skin-care products called Le Mirador. But I never set out solely to have great skin. I owe my appearance to my health, and I owe my health to one decision: to eat my food raw. It was a necessary decision with some very pleasant, added benefits. In addition to transforming my health and having a positive effect on my appearance, eating raw has made me feel amazing.

I always feel satisfied—something very few people, much less models, can say. I feel happy and healthy, and I am. I feel a sense of there being a great deal of variety in my life and a quality of abundance I didn't know before. I feel beautiful and youthful in a way that I didn't when I was much younger and eating all the dead garbage that most of us eat. I feel creative, innovative, clearer, and, yes, different in a way that lets me know I'm doing something for myself that isn't ordinary, run-of-the-mill, or boring. Eating raw just feels right.

And it shows. People remark that they sense a vitality in me that they didn't in the days before I began eating this way. They see a life in me that they didn't see before because, in fact, it wasn't there before.

Eating is now exciting for me every day and I'm *never hungry*.

For anyone in the public eye, and especially anyone who makes their living in large part based on how they appear, eating tends to loom large in life. It becomes more than something you do to satisfy (or sadly, not satisfy) a hunger. Because your diet can determine what you weigh, how you look, how you feel, and the image you convey, it all too easily can become a focal point of your life.

Models and actors are dogged by the food they consume. Many diet incessantly. And the world follows, yearning to have the abs of so-and-so or the butt of what's-her-name.

I'm one of the fortunate few who no longer find themselves struggling, and I thank God for that. I never worry about whether I should eat or not. I never skip a meal, I never crave food, and I never feel guilty for eating.

Before eating raw I was sick a lot. I mean I really didn't feel well. I struggled with the chronic, bothersome health issues that most people think are normal. We simply pop a pill and go on our way. I had acid indigestion all the time and ate Tums like candy. I had headaches two or three times a week. My sinuses were a mess. The fear of colds and flu plagued me. The list goes on and on.

Since I started eating raw, all these problems have cleared up. I'm healthier than ever. I rarely if ever get sick. And I look different. Without trying to, I look and feel better, healthier, and younger than I did when I was eating cooked

comes into contact with oxygen in the air and the oxidation process begins, chemically changing the juice and neutralizing certain vitamins. That's why you should drink fresh juice pretty quickly. Even in the refrigerator the oxygen rapidly depletes the nutritional value of fruits and vegetables. Still, even with all these limitations, eating fresh is always best!

# the raw debate:
## vegetarian or not?

A lot of raw foodists and alternative-food proponents in general treat everyone the same, and think everyone should be eating the same foods. But people come from a variety of environmental and genetic backgrounds. When you look at anthropological literature, there is no escaping the truth of humans having inhabited a variety of ecological niches. As a result, different people need different foods for optimal health. I may dream of living in a tropical paradise, but my ancestors come from—and I live somewhere—very different. Humans always have and probably always will live in places as different as the perennially frozen Arctic, the equatorial jungles, and everywhere in between. As a result, we have eaten very different diets. That is, until the last several decades, when preserving food and transporting it across half the world has become common. Now we have become pretty homogenized.

It used to be that we ate whatever we could get locally and in season. The Eskimo who live in the Arctic were classic meat eaters, and people in the rain forest were principally vegetarians. The traditional Eskimo diet was well studied at the beginning of the twentieth century by Vilhjalmur Stefansson and the great Arctic explorers, and it was established that their diet was about 20 percent protein and 80 percent fat. Of course, in the Arctic Circle there is no growing season, there is no soil to till, and there are no sources of fruits, nuts, seeds, or grain. When the traditional Eskimo were eating the traditional meat diet, they were among the healthiest people that had been studied anywhere—with no heart disease, low cholesterol, low arteriosclerosis, and none of the degenerative diseases from which much of the world suffers. However, when the Eskimos

went into the towns and cities and began eating a lower-fat diet, a Western diet of breakfast cereals and junk food, they started to get obese and they developed the degenerative diseases that plague them today. The famous Masai in Kenya, and the Nuer and Dinka from the Sudan, for example, have a largely milk-blood diet in which most of their calories come from animal protein. It's an extraordinarily high saturated-fat diet, and yet these traditional peoples are unusually healthy.

The idea that humans are vegetarian by nature simply isn't validated by anthropological literature. Not only do we have the teeth of omnivores—those who eat a mixed plant- and meat-based diet—but even today the Eskimos are people who really need to eat red meat to be healthy. A study published in the *New England Journal of Medicine* showed that Eskimos lack some of the enzymes needed to break down cooked complex carbohydrates—something they never developed because they never used to eat our "well-rounded diet." No complex carbohydrates grow in the far northern reaches of North America. So if they eat white sugar (which in my view isn't good for anyone!) or even whole grains, they're not going to do well. Eskimo cell metabolism requires fat to produce energy; they don't produce it from carbohydrates very effectively. They actually need saturated fat, and they thrive on it.

On the other hand, if you go to the equatorial regions—the Amazon, for example—you'll find peoples who eat largely a plant-based diet, and they derive sufficient proteins from it. It's estimated that some of the North American Indians east of the Mississippi knew of a thousand edible plants and, like the Amazonian Indians, they lived principally off the vegetation. And they did so very efficiently and were traditionally very healthy. But further west, the Plains Indians largely lived off the buffalo herds—very successfully. So even within North America there was a great variation in indigenous diets.

So I'm not an across-the-board proponent of a raw, strictly plant-based diet for everyone. I have no doubt it's right for some people, but it may not be (and probably isn't) right for everyone. My boyfriend is an athlete. He's originally from Russia. He's extraordinarily healthy and eats mostly raw foods. But what does he crave? Red meat. And he eats a lot of it. I occasionally eat meat too, as well as fish and dairy; I just eat it mostly raw. When I was first introduced to eating raw by Dr. Brantley, the question of possibly becoming a vegetarian or a

vegan never came up. Only recently have I met more and more raw vegans whose philosophy of life opposes humans consuming animal products. It seems that many, if not most, of the prominent raw foodists are vegans. I can't speak for them. But I do share the concern that many of them express over the torture of animals who become our food. It's important, therefore, to seek out organic, free-range meat to ensure that the animals were properly treated.

# benefits of
## eating raw

Unlike the millions of people who deprive themselves on diets, I eat as much as I want—so long as it's raw. I don't limit myself to one piece of raw coconut pie or thirty germinated almonds or any other measured serving. If I want to eat more, I do. I don't count raw calories or raw fat grams. I don't calculate how much of a given raw food I might eat. I don't weigh anything. That's something I let my body dictate. What freedom!

At age thirty-two, when I was eating cooked food, I was starving myself yet still had trouble keeping extra weight off. Now in my forties, I eat what I want— but just raw—and maintain my weight without even trying to. If anything, I may have trouble keeping weight on because I'm almost never hungry and always satisfied when I eat. I don't walk away from the table still wishing I could have more. I walk away full, satisfied, without thinking about what I wish I could have eaten but had to sacrifice to stay in model/actress form.

Our society is beset with obesity. It is a growing problem, even in kids, but it is something that becomes more and more of a problem as people age. It doesn't take someone who eats raw food to see that the obesity problem is reaching epidemic proportions. I'm struck that there are very few overweight raw foodists, young or old. But there are lots of them who are trim and beautiful and look younger than their years—or at least more beautiful and younger than many others their age who eat cooked food and seem to be aging prematurely.

And what about beauty? Though we women would like to pretend that we're flawless (or at least magazines present models that way), I confess I'm not. In

case there are any men reading this, pay attention: most women have some cellulite, models and actresses included (sorry, guys, I really do hate to ruin the illusion). Most magazine photos are *retouched!* (However, the cover of this book is not!)

Here's a confession: I have never liked to work out, and I really don't have a strict regimen I stick to. Okay, I'm an exercise slacker (and I'm not saying you should be). But there was a time, back in my cooked-food days, when slacking off at the gym meant I would suffer the consequences in a serious way. There was no way I could go for two days without doing my five hundred sit-ups because *it would show.* Now, when I work out I see changes faster, and muscle tone and definition last longer. I have better ab definition now without even trying than I ever did before. I don't want to leave you with the wrong impression—it didn't happen overnight. But I recently realized that one of the cumulative effects of eating raw over these years is that I have lost the fat and there is muscle where I could never quite see it, even though I worked out all those years. There's almost a six-pack where before there was a suck-it-in layer of fat. So I strongly believe in the positive effects eating raw can have on staying toned.

Critics of eating raw foods often assume something must be missing in a raw diet. Some think eating raw will make you sick. For me in fact, since eating raw I no longer suffer from the headaches, heartburn, colds, flu, allergies, or sinus problems that once seemed to plague me. And my overall mood has changed. I'm no longer sluggish, and I don't lack desire for work or sex.

I'm amazed sometimes at how some people care a lot about how they look but don't really care about their health. Maybe I have been eating raw for too long to recall what it was like *not* to make the connection among health, the appearance of beauty, and true vitality. But it makes sense to me that if you *are* healthy you'll *look* healthy. And if you look healthy you'll look younger. Vitality and youth go hand in hand. So it should come as no surprise that if there is a fountain of youth to be found it's as close to you as what you put into your body and how it is prepared. And if you have to choose between consuming dead food that your body has to reprocess or living food that provides you with what you need to sustain and foster life, well, I prefer life over death and the living over the dying. And people tell me it shows. I've already told you how I can see

the difference in my skin. The same is true for my hair, and even my eyes are different. Eating raw, the whites are whiter and the blue got lighter.

I do look younger. My skin is more supple now and I have fewer wrinkles than I did before eating raw. I remember the day my mother, who can be my most loving but honest critic, came up to me and told me that she couldn't believe how my skin had changed. Of course, I'm not the only one. I believe you see the change in people when they switch over from cooked to raw food and it only grows with time. I see it a lot in the raw foodists I meet. There is a youthful appearance and a happiness. They simply look better.

The proof *is* in the proverbial (yes, uncooked) pudding—*and that doesn't mean just Carol Alt.* I have seen it in the health and beauty and wellness of countless raw foodists, women and men from all walks of life who, whether they understand exactly how raw foods nourish them or not, have been able to experience a vitality they never imagined was possible.

You could be one of us.

# 4 what is raw?

## calling things what they are

If you've read the previous chapters, you've heard my story. You know how and why I began eating raw, how it has changed my life, and what pleasure and satisfaction it has brought me. As a result, if you're not already into raw food, I hope you're at least beginning to understand the benefits of eating this way. You already have some ideas about what raw food is. If nothing more, you know that raw food is uncooked! That's a start. But we haven't really discussed the question what *is* raw food? ✳ The answer seems simple enough but,

in fact, not all uncooked foods—not even uncooked foods of the same kind—are created equal. One uncooked cauliflower is not as good for you as the next. Since not everyone who eats raw agrees about what to eat and what not to eat, let me begin to explain.

Different people will say different things about what is raw and what is not. Strictly speaking, any form of alteration, adulteration, depletion, or transformation of a food that diminishes its original nutritional content or modifies its living structure makes it less than "truly raw." But we live in an imperfect world. I accept that. My standard for food is this: the *more* living, fresh, organic, and uncooked a food is, the better! Dr. Brantley once told me that the closer I eat to God—meaning from the earth to me with no one in between cooking, X-raying, homogenizing, and so forth—the better it is for me. I like to think that when it comes to what we put into our bodies, we should take the ancient Greek father of medicine, Hippocrates, seriously and "first do no harm." But why just avoid harm? Why not do good too? I want the best food my body can find. Here are some factors to look out for as you start exploring the world of raw food.

# irradiation

Some raw foods are intrinsically more desirable—meaning they're better in nutritional quality and more "life giving"—than others. Cooking isn't the only thing that damages food. Today many foods, without our being told, are being "irradiated." A food that is irradiated isn't cooked in the traditional sense, but it is processed in a way that alters the molecular structure and the integrity of food. It is hit with radiation. I believe it is no longer life giving in the same way that a natural, unadulterated food is. You'll hear all sorts of things about how irradiation is harmless. But supposedly so is cooking. How does irradiation work? There are three different kinds of irradiation technology. One exposes foods to a radioactive substance, either cobalt or cesium. Another streams high-energy electrons into the food. The third zaps food with X-rays. Each kills supposedly disease-causing microorganisms even though a certain amount of the right soil organism is actually good for you. At the same time they kill essential

life-giving enzymes and nutrients. Speaking for myself, if food is irradiated I want nothing to do with it.

# preservatives

Similarly, salad greens that are soaked in preservatives such as sulfites to keep them crisp and colorful on the salad bar (or even in the produce section of your supermarket) are raw from the standpoint of cooking. But while they appear fresh for a long time, they simply aren't. It's all show. They have more in common with a well-made-up embalmed veggie corpse than live, organic raw food. They can cause liver toxicity and elicit severe allergic-like reactions in sensitive people. I can't honestly consider preservative-filled foods raw.

When I say I want fresh food, I mean food that is still living. Preservatives are out, period. Substances that were formerly foods but have turned into potential museum exhibits simply are not food. That means no MSG (monosodium glutamate), no BHA (butylated hydroxyanisole) or BHT (butylated hydroxytoluene). No sodium nitrite, sodium sulfite, or sodium dioxide. These chemicals are *not* welcome in my kitchen, let alone in my body. (Read the labels on most dried fruits!)

Canned foods are never fresh, and most have preservatives in them. Even if they don't contain preservatives, they are nearly always cooked before being canned. And whether they are cooked or not, keeping something in a can on a shelf for a long time requires that the enzymes be destroyed so that the food would be dead, and if the food's not dead I don't want to know what might be alive and growing inside!

# pesticides

Fresh-picked foods sprayed with pesticides or grown in soils that have been depleted of their mineral content may be raw in the sense that they are uncooked, but they too are far less than ideal as foods because they might contain potentially dangerous chemical additives or have been robbed of essential

nutrients that your body craves. And what about foods that have been genetically altered? That's a subject worthy of a whole book. But let's just say this: perhaps we should take a hint from the Europeans, who will not import American foods that have been altered genetically or have been injected with hormones. They consider these foods to be a significant health risk.

# fresh
## food

For a food to be living, it has to be fresh. Whenever any food is harvested it begins to lose its vitality. Some foods are naturally protected from the air, and their vitality is captured, slowing down the process of spoiling. The peel on a banana, for example, is virtually airtight. It's nature's attempt at keeping the fruit's nutritious contents fresh for as long as possible. Remove the peel and expose it to air, and you better eat it or it will turn brown and rapidly start to spoil. Bananas travel well. If they didn't, we wouldn't get them in North America. Some other foods don't stay fresh nearly as long. Meat and fish, for example, deteriorate very quickly, and even some fruits and vegetables such as mineral-dense lettuces last only a few days in prime condition after being picked.

Since the beginning of time, humans have tried to preserve food from the ravages of time and the changes of seasons. In recent history, we have developed refrigeration, freezing, and vacuum sealing—the three best ways to keep many foods fresh for as long as possible. But not all of these methods are good for all foods. A frozen banana may in itself be delicious, but have you ever seen what one looks and tastes like after it is thawed? Trust me, while it may be the next best thing to a ripe, truly fresh banana in terms of nutrition, it looks and tastes nothing like a fresh banana—or anything the vast majority of us would want to eat.

Thankfully, fresh foods are readily available almost everywhere today. (For a starter list of places where you might find some, check out chapter 6.) As a general rule, Dr. Brantley once told me that if you can't find the top ten items on your shopping list in the two outermost aisles of the supermarket—where you

find the fresh produce and the meat and fish departments—you're not buying raw food. And even there, you may not be choosing the best examples of raw foods that you could find if you make some extra effort.

# organic
## food

The economics of producing food has created a trade-off between what is most nutritious and what produces the highest yield and most reliable crop. To succeed in the highly competitive world of agriculture, farmers put artificial pesticides, herbicides, and fertilizers into soils. It's not good for the soil, it's not good for the food, and it's not good for you and me. But it is good for business because it keeps food costs down and profits predictable. As a result, there's a lot of produce out there in the stores that looks good but could be a lot better for you (and taste better too) if it weren't for the power and profit making of big business. Let's hear it for laissez-faire capitalism!

It's hard to believe that just a century ago this was not so. But the development of chemicals and technologies for warfare in World Wars I and II spawned the agri-chemical business and with it came the use of DDT (dichlorodiphenyl-trichloroethane) as a way to kill insects in 1939. DDT has since been banned in the United States, but parathion, an organophosphorous pesticide developed in 1943, is still used today. So are countless other synthetic substances. And while produce exposed to DDT is not supposed to be imported into the United States, some does slip through.

There was a time when farming was organic. Organic agriculture is the oldest form of agriculture on earth. Instead of using artificial chemical fertilizers and pesticides, organic farmers rotate and cover crops and use natural-based products to maintain soils and increase their fertility. They allow fields to lie fallow, to "rest." They use natural means to limit the growth of pests and increase the populations of beneficial insects (yes, there are "good bugs"). As a result, the food you get is not laced with chemicals that can make you sick. It is organic (natural, or living) as opposed to inorganic (artificial, or dead).

It seems like a pretty simple concept to me: "healthy soil, healthy food, healthy people"—which is also the slogan of the Rodale Institute, associated with Rodale Press, the health-and-fitness publisher. If we are principally concerned about people (and not just profits) we should promote the production and consumption of healthy food, and the healthiest foods come from healthy soils. In stores such as Whole Foods Market and Wild Oats, the produce is marked either "conventional" or "organic." If I have a choice, I buy foods that are organic. While they're not putting the major supermarket chains out of business, more and more Whole Foods Market and Wild Oats stores and others like them are opening all across the United States and in Canada. You can find the one nearest to you through their Web sites, www.wholefoods.com and www.wildoats.com. But even if there isn't one near you, it's still possible to find smaller local supermarkets and health-food stores that carry organic foods. Call around and ask the health-food stores. Just be very picky and careful about your raw sources.

# uncooked
## food

Okay, this seems obvious—raw food is uncooked food. In the United States, by law, raw foods should be clearly marked with terms such as raw, cold-pressed, *unpasteurized, crude, crue,* uncooked, unprocessed, and so on. That's pretty simple. But the problem is that there are all sorts of cooked foods masquerading as raw. These include various dairy products. If something is pasteurized, it is cooked. You won't find raw milk in the dairy section (in most places, it's actually against the law). And unless your supermarket has an excellent cheese selection and is serious about marking the raw ones, you'll have to spend some time looking at labels to identify the ones that aren't pasteurized or have additives. (It's amazing what you'll find in the cheese section, including some things labeled "cheese product"—meaning they aren't really cheese at all!) Generally speaking, unless it's found in the produce section of the store or bought directly from the farm, raw food must say "raw." If it doesn't, it is nearly certain that what you have is not raw.

Canned foods are almost certain to be cooked. That canned tuna is not raw. Forget canned vegetables. Even if they bear some resemblance to fresh, uncooked food, they're not. They're cooked.

Take lox, for example. Though it looks a lot like sliced, fresh salmon, lox is *smoked* salmon and, yes, *smoking is cooking.* But in some stores right next to the lox in the same sort of packaging you'll find salmon slices in marinades or cured with salt, and these can be considered raw. (My favorite kind is Spence & Company gravlax.) So it's not always so easy to tell cooked from uncooked food at first glance. It's important to actually read the label to see how things are prepared. It may take awhile, but you'll begin to get very good at figuring out which foods are cooked and which are not because they are side by side. It's just a matter of practice, and once you know you'll keep coming back for your favorite products.

The temperature at which food is served is not a reliable indicator of whether something is raw or cooked. Of course, if food is steaming hot you know it is cooked. But there are gazpachos that are served cold but are made with canned tomatoes that are definitely cooked. There are cold pasta salads that are made from cooked wheat, something I won't even consider eating. And the hummus you'll find in your local supermarket has cooked chickpeas even though it's kept refrigerated. Then again, there are raw pastas, such as the Spaghetti al Pesto (page 150) and Raw Hummus (page 142) in chapter 10 that are neither made from wheat nor served chilled (they're served at room temperature).

# mixed
## foods

One restaurant I frequent in New York is Sushi Samba. The tuna and salmon seviches there are among my favorite main courses, and that's why these recipes are also in this book. Along with their various kinds of sashimi, you couldn't ask for more delicious, high-protein raw foods anywhere.

Seviche and sashimi are raw foods but sushi itself is *not.* That's right—though

it is served cold, sushi is typically made from a combination of various uncooked, sashimi-grade seafoods and *cooked* white rice. Since rice is hard and undigestible when it's uncooked, the only way to eat it raw is to germinate it, which they don't do at most non-raw restaurants. So give me the fish but spare me the rice.

One of the most common misconceptions people have about eating raw food is that it's really all about salads, which is wrong on two fronts. First, as you already know by now, there is a lot more to eat without cooking than lettuce and veggies in a bowl. But equally wrong is the notion that anything you find in a salad is raw. Like sushi, many salads are mixed foods, partially raw and partially cooked. For example, if you have a hard-boiled egg in a salad, it's cooked. If you add dressing, there is a good chance that it's made, either partially or fully, from cooked ingredients. I am not saying you can *never* eat anything that is cooked. What I am saying is that a lot of raw foods come with cooked foods, and you should be aware of that. And, as with sushi, even if the food on your plate seems raw, you should be honest with yourself and recognize that you're eating a mixed food.

# vegetarian, vegan, and raw foods

It's also important to make some distinctions among vegetarian, vegan, and raw food. When people hear that I eat raw food, many assume I'm a vegetarian. I'm not. The fact is that more and more, I'm inclined to pass on eating meat. But I do eat raw dairy products and some raw fish if I find a reliable source. The day may come when I give up eating these things entirely, and then I will be a raw vegetarian.

There are many raw foodists who are vegetarians, and a good number are not only vegetarians but go one step further and become vegans. A vegan diet not only excludes animal flesh but all other animal products as well. This means no eggs, no dairy, and in some circles even no honey since it is an animal prod-

uct; most vegans cook their food. But most of the best-known figures in the raw-food movement eat a raw-vegan diet. My favorite raw restaurants do not serve meat, fish, eggs, milk, or cheese. Some serve honey. They are considered raw-vegan restaurants.

There are a number of reasons people choose one or another of the possible forms of raw foodism. I started eating raw for health reasons. Many start out with health concerns that lead them to associate with people whose worldview includes other ethical issues and philosophies. While I am a spiritually sensitive person, my own religious background and moral convictions have meant I've never so much as flirted with Eastern religious philosophies or practices where dietary practices and prohibitions are spelled out explicitly. Many who follow this route become vegetarian or vegan. Not me. Besides, there are essential nutrients and oils that are more readily available in meats, fish, and dairy than they are in vegetables.

# keeping
# kosher

Quintessence Restaurant, my regular haunt in New York, serves vegan food but allows honey products. And while probably only a very few of its patrons think of it as anything but a raw restaurant, in fact all of its food is also kosher. Not being Jewish, eating kosher food isn't essential to me. But even for the non-observant there is something to be said for traditional dietary regulations. I don't eat bottom-dwelling seafood, for example, and if it comes out of the water but doesn't have fins (unless it's a sea vegetable) I won't touch it. Nevertheless, anyone who wants to keep kosher should know that it's possible to eat both raw and kosher. Recipes in the book like Spaghetti al Pesto (page 150), Carol's Everyday Guacamole (page 141) and countless utterly scrumptious desserts prove that indeed it's "easy as (raw) pie."

# 5

# starting raw

**beginners' steps on the raw adventure**

How you get started eating raw depends a lot on your temperament and personality. ✳ My boyfriend went cold turkey. One day he just decided to go for it and switched over from cooked food to raw rood. He never went back. But then many elite competitive athletes are that way— it's all or nothing. Simply by deciding, he became a raw foodist virtually overnight. ✳ For me, it was more gradual. My first conversation with the brilliant Dr. Brantley made me start paying attention to exactly what it was that I was putting into my body. (Looking back now on

what I used to eat, I have to wonder: What was I thinking? Was I suicidal?) I started to take an inventory of what I had been eating. I made incremental changes by cutting things out of my diet and introducing others, and before long I was eating almost 90–95 percent raw. But it didn't happen overnight. I started to eat raw bit by bit, and in the end it has had a tremendous impact on my life and my health—and it did so quickly. I would never turn back.

# ten steps
## to raw

If you're not the all-or-nothing type but more gradual like me, I'd love to share with you how you can experience the pleasure and reap the benefits of raw food. Here's what helped me change my life, in ten simple steps:

## 1. search your memory

Sit down and take a mental inventory of what you ate over the last three days. You can't change what you have already eaten so just be honest. Include every-thing. This includes snacks and anything you happened to put in to your mouth. Remember, be honest.

## 2. make a list

Take note of what foods you toss into your mouth over the next three days and what time you eat it. Write it down. Keep the list with you and add to it, day by day. Just doing this will begin to make you more keenly aware of specifically what it is you eat and when—and that awareness is key. Once you know what you eat and when you eat it, you'll start to be more empowered to make changes. As you do this, feel free to eat more raw foods starting right now.

## 3. identify the raw

Once you have your list, think about what foods I have mentioned that you already eat raw—those that you already have in your diet. Maybe you didn't eat them in the last week but you like them. For example, perhaps you like seared

steak or eat your steak "black and blue." The "blue" is 100 percent raw food. Perhaps you like seared tuna and you eat it whenever you find it on the menu. Maybe you are a salad nut. Perhaps you love berries or bananas or California oranges. Good for you. This is the beginning of eating raw. Some people already have a lengthy list of raw foods they like, while others (like me when I started) have nearly none. Whatever your case may be, it's a starting point, and don't sell it short. Start where you are, with what you already know, feel comfortable with, and enjoy.

## 4. find a lost twin

Now, look at your favorite foods and think about which ones may have a raw twin. For example, you may like cheese (and you may not eat cheese because it is "fattening"). Well, hallelujah! You can add some cheese back into your diet if you'll go that extra inch and ask for "raw-milk cheeses" at your local cheese store or Whole Foods Market. Maybe you like salsa or guacamole. If you make it fresh and skip the canned or jarred varieties, then it is raw. (There are recipes for both of them right here in this book.) If you like bagels with lox for breakfast, replace the smoked salmon with "gravlax" salmon, which is just as tasty but is sometimes marinated rather than smoked (which, of course, means cooked). Replace the cream cheese with a raw Camembert and you've transformed everything but the bagel. Then switch over to Ezekiel bread instead—even though it's not 100 percent raw, it is still better for you because it is baked at low temperatures and made from sprouted grains. There are countless ways to use raw honey instead of sugar or sugar substitutes (which are all chemicals) that you have probably never considered.

## 5. look at the "raw day"

Now let's look at how you eat throughout your day as a whole. Say you're used to three meals a day. Set your sights on eating a 2-to-1 ratio of raw to cooked meals and you should have a pretty easy transition. I suggest making breakfast and lunch the mostly raw meals and dinner the mostly cooked meal. I recommend this for a number of reasons.

Breakfast is what fuels us during the day when we need to think and work. Lunch keeps that energy flowing through the day. Though we tend to make it

more important than breakfast or lunch, dinner is actually much less important to our energy levels because we usually go to bed shortly thereafter. So late in the day, what do you need so much raw energy for? (Okay, maybe there is more to life in the raw than just eating, working, and sleeping!) For most people who are just getting started, I suggest eating rice (maybe a risotto for instance) with a salad or other raw mixture of veggies for dinner the first two months to help transition to raw, because with so much white flour in the American diet (and many other diets for that matter) nearly every person in the country has issues with sugar/starch addiction. It's a hard thing for many people to over-come. So do like Dr. Brantley did with me: Eat two meals a day as raw as you can and then eat potatoes or whole grains like rice or quinoa (no wheat flour) with lightly cooked vegetables or a salad for dinner. Then after two months, decide you're going to transition off of this routine to eat as much raw at each meal—including dinner—as you can. It may sound impossible now, but in a couple months it won't be. In fact, you may find you've done it in much less time than that.

## 6. consider each meal

As you begin eating raw, look at each meal separately and not just what you eat over the course of the day as a whole. Each meal is a unique opportunity to prepare something nutritious for the body, so that's why you should try to cre-ate each meal on the same 2-to-1 ratio of raw and cooked—eating two-thirds raw food and one-third cooked food. If you like steak and eggs for breakfast, choose a larger portion of organic steak and sear it and have only one egg. At least the meat will be mostly raw. Or try Spence & Co. instead of lox with a small salad with cold-pressed oil. For lunch, order your steak, tuna, or fish lightly seared. Eat a healthy salad topped with a handful of germinated chickpeas. Spread raw-milk cheese onto Ezekiel bread, and top with sprouts or ripe tomatoes.

So here's a summary so far: You continue to eat the raw foods that you already like. You look at the cooked food you like and try to find raw substitutes. Then you eat two meals each day, preferably breakfast and lunch, eating as much of the meals raw as is possible. Easy enough.

Okay, let's move on . . .

# 7. name your exceptions

This step was crucial to me: identify the foods that you love cooked and can't find raw, and decide how many times a month you "need" to eat these. I have many friends and family who said to me, "I can't eat raw because I love pasta" or "I can't do this because I love Thai food." I think that's fair. But ask yourself how many times a month you "need" pasta? Once, twice, weekly perhaps? And can you at least find a pasta that has no wheat flour? Could you replace it with a rice pasta or spelt or kamut? Now you're making intelligent choices. Make an occasional rice pasta your "cheat," your exception, instead of one made from wheat flour with its gluten. And what about that Thai food? Well, it turns out that my friend who simply couldn't imagine living without it really only ate it once every now and then anyway. He simply needed to know he had the option of tasting it from time to time and didn't want his "choice" taken away. Well, whatever rings your chimes. Knowing you can have something you love to eat when you want it really makes you want it less.

Don't go overboard, but do allow yourself to have exceptions—specifically *your* exceptions. But be sure to identify them. Name them. Then you'll be able to eat them guilt-free—occasionally.

When I started eating raw, my big thing was nacho chips. Just simply couldn't live without them (or so I thought). So I made them my cheat. They were the food I would "binge" on once a week and eventually twice a month. I just ate them when I absolutely, positively had to have them. And those moments became fewer and fewer. I didn't suffer without them. And now I wonder what I needed them so desperately for. Of course, I still have a little popcorn at hockey games.

# 8. avoid hunger

Breakfast really is the most important meal of the day, so get used to treating it that way. Remind yourself that without your breakfast your body has nothing to run on. If your body has nothing to run on, then when you run out of gas, you'll eat whatever is available without thinking. Why do you think candy companies are a 100 billion-dollar-a-year worldwide business? It might happen at eleven in the morning or it might happen at four in the afternoon, but it does happen to everyone. Don't let it happen to you.

So let's talk about breakfast. Many people avoid the first meal of the day because it's not a social meal; this is a big mistake. When I was starting out eating raw I would go out to dinner and order salad, fish, and rice. I ate the rice and half the salad for dinner but took the rest home for breakfast. Fish and salad in the morning? You bet! If that combination first thing in the morning sounds strange to you, remember lox with lettuce on a bagel? The reason I brought home my breakfast was that I was too lazy to get up really early and make something to eat to start my day. I wanted it there, ready to eat or to take to the office. If you're the type of person who will get up and fix her breakfast, get in the habit of making it raw. If you're not, then remember to get whatever you like to eat ready the night before so it's ready to go. Go to chapter 10 and make David Wolfe's Basic Breakfast Granola (page 127) with Juliano's Whipped Cream (page 157), for example.

But what about lunch? Early on I got into the habit of bringing my own raw-milk cheeses to work with me and added them to salads, along with sprouted breads, seared steak, sashimi-grade fish, whatever I could find already made in the restaurant or anything else raw that was already familiar to me. That way I could instantly create a satisfying raw meal and wouldn't be tempted by non-raw options. Snacks? I carried germinated mixed nuts and dried fruits for a ready made "trail mix."

# 9. go hunting

Get out of your usual food shopping rut. In chapter 6 you will learn about all the places you could be shopping for the foods that you really want to eat. Make it a fun social thing to do with friends. Break the old supermarket habit and replace it with new ways to hunt for and find raw foods. Once you figure out where to "stalk" them, there will be an abundance of raw food on your table.

# 10. add, change, become

As you learn where to find what you want and what you like and don't like (because like cooked food, we each have things we prefer and things we don't), you will be able to add more and more from the cornucopia of raw possibilities to what you actually eat. Change is always difficult at first, but, frankly, the benefits make it easy. Besides, you'll be amazed at the possibilities, and the tastes

will surprise and delight you. Become the healthy, beautiful raw person you can be. Before long you'll wonder how you ever did anything else.

"This is about abundance, not deprivation," says David Wolfe, an authority on raw food. He's absolutely right. But for most people it's a gradual process. The cleaner your body gets, the more it will prefer raw food. Believe me, you will know the difference because you will begin to feel bad after eating cooked food. Your body will naturally pick the food it needs most and likes best, and raw food will become your body's food of choice. You probably won't miss cooked food (or the usual heartburn that goes along with it). The abundance from eating raw is positively seductive.

# balancing
## your raw diet

As you begin to explore the world of eating raw, it's important to make sure that you are eating a healthy mix of different types of raw foods, including proteins, carbohydrates, healthy fats, and, of course, healthy portions of vitamin- and mineral-dense fruits and vegetables. Keep this in mind as you plan out your meals and begin getting into the rhythm of eating raw. When I started out, my friend and mentor, Timothy Brantley, ND, always reminded me to eat a wide variety of foods.

You should have fats, long-chain carbohydrates, and proteins at each meal. Yes, you can have raw, sprouted legumes instead of meats for your protein (Dr. Brantley told me cooked legumes like lentil soup or storebought hummus are actually carbohydrates). Have vegetable salads (which are long-chain carbohydrates) instead of baked breads (short-chain carbs). "Eat the colors of the rainbow in your salad, a wide spectrum" of vegetables, Dr. Timothy always says. You should have at least a tablespoon of fat at each meal, so don't spare the cold-pressed olive oil. Of course you can also get your fat in raw cheese or hummus, for example. For a basic well-rounded meal have a seared steak, salad, and sprouted bread. But the possibilities are many.

As you plan your meals, keep these staples in mind:

✳ **Proteins.** These include germinated nuts, sprouted seeds, raw cheeses, and raw or lightly seared meat and fish.

✳ **Long-chain carbohydrates.** These include sprouted grains and sprouted grain breads and vegetables.

✳ **Healthy fats.** These include avocados, coconuts, and cold-pressed oils.

# supplements
## for the raw-food eater

Whatever food it happens to be, I always try to get it in the most nutritious, natural state—raw. But in this day and age, even if you're eating certified organic food, the soils aren't as good as they were one hundred years ago. Acid rain dumps pollutants even on organic farms. As a result, there's no such thing as perfect food anymore. We make do with the best we can get. I think E3 Live™ or green powders are great in general as supplemental nutrition. They provide whole nutrients in a much more usable form than typical vitamin supplements.

Theoretically, no one should have to take supplements. When people hear I eat raw, they often wonder whether I take supplements. They'll say, "If you're eating a natural diet you shouldn't have to take supplements." In a perfect world, they'd be absolutely correct. But even the organic foods from our soils aren't as good as they once were and as they should be. There's acid rain even in the Arctic Circle. Not one spot on the entire earth is completely free from the toxins that, once they enter our bodies, need to be neutralized—something we're surprisingly good at. But at a cost. And if the day comes that the world is made perfect again, none of the raw foodists will have to take supplements. (Notice I said *raw foodists.* Those who eat cooked food mostly will likely still suffer the same consequences that they do now.) Meanwhile, I take all-natural, organic, powdered supplements (as opposed to tablets or caplets). If I eat any cooked food, I also take enzymes. I've found Quantum Nutrition Labs "Digest" or Dr. Timothy Brantley's Premier Enzymes work best for me. But supplements are just that: they supplement what should be available to us in our food.

# 6

## getting fresh

### where you can find what you need and want

When I started eating raw eight years ago, it took some serious work to make or find the food I needed for a well-rounded diet of fresh, raw foods. I'm happy to report that things have become dramatically easier since then. With markets that specialize in fresh, organic foods, and Internet sites to order anything you can't find locally, eating raw and being thoroughly satisfied is now pretty simple. But even back when I was just beginning, it wasn't impossible if you knew where to go and what to get. ✳ I could have written this

chapter for all the fortunate people in California who have every raw resource imaginable right around the corner—all right, maybe a few miles down the freeway. But that's too easy. Besides, most people don't live in LA, and very few of us have everything we could possibly want right at our fingertips. Because I'm convinced that anyone anywhere should be able to and can eat raw, I'm going to explain how to get what you need the way I did when I started out in Santa Monica in 1996. That was before Southern California became what it is today—the raw-food mecca that lures pilgrims from the ends of the earth.

The things I consume are infinitely more imaginative and enticing than a bowl of greens followed by a piece of fruit for dessert. But as with preparing cooked food, to make something that's truly safe, healthy, and satisfying you have to know where to get what you need. That's what this chapter will try to help you with.

# local
# supermarket

It's hard for some committed raw foodists to imagine, but when I began eating raw the local supermarket was the main place to shop—just as it still is for people in Peoria and Detroit and Great Falls. And you might be surprised by how many raw options are available there.

## produce

When Timothy Brantley told me that if it's not in the first two outer aisles, you probably don't want it, my view of the supermarket produce aisle quickly changed—out of necessity. Fruits and vegetables I had walked past and never really noticed before suddenly seemed to stand out. Thai coconuts. Avocados. Cilantro. It's not as though I never knew they existed. I never knew how to use them and how versatile they were, so I just never paid much attention to them. For many of you, now is the time for you to take note of the wide variety of nutritious living foods you've been walking past all these years. Yes, even eating raw you'll probably still only eat some of them. But this is where to start—noticing what it is you have been missing.

If you look at some of the recipes in this book, you'll see there is a wide array of nutritious fresh fruits and vegetables that appear over and over in recipe after recipe. One of these is the avocado. Far from being used only in guacamole—the most common way Americans know avocados—its subtle and adaptable flavor invites use in lots of recipes. How many people would think of avocados as a principal ingredient in a mouthwateringly delicious and nutritious, no-guilt dessert mousse? Until I started eating raw, it never would have occurred to me, and until I tasted it, the thought had turned me off.

The produce section of your supermarket is *the* place to start as you begin eating raw. In this book's recipes alone you'll find strawberries and other berries, bananas, pears, apples, watermelon, lemons, and limes. There are mushrooms, cauliflower, red and green cabbage, carrots, zucchini, shallots, red and green bell peppers, cucumbers, celery, tomatoes, romaine lettuce, scallions, garlic, white and red onions, and mesclun greens. In addition to fresh herbs such as basil, oregano, tarragon, rosemary, parsley, cilantro, sage, and dill, you'll find Thai coconuts, gingerroot, dates, jalapeño peppers, and, of course, avocados. And all these ingredients don't just make great salads—they make great soups, sauces, and desserts.

If you ask me, that's a lot from the produce department!

Not every supermarket will stock every one of these items, but most of them are there. You may not have seen them before, but if you look, chances are you'll find them. If not, it's worth asking the produce managers if and when they can get what you're looking for. Be sure to ask for organic versions of your favorite produce.

## pure water

Besides fresh produce there are other staples in the raw kitchen that you can find at the supermarket. The most obvious is water. Yes, water. Pure, fresh, clean water. This is one of the absolute essentials we often overlook because we have grown up with what we believe to be fresh water. I admit, compared with many places in the world, our water is relatively safe. When you consider that in Haiti, barely a few hundred miles from American soil, the principal causes of death are no water, bad water, no food, and bad food (dehydration, dysentery, starvation, and malnutrition), we can be thankful that our tap water is drinkable! But

it is still not truly good for you. What you need if you want to be healthy is water that is not just free of pesky microorganisms that can cause stomach cramps, fever, and the runs. It should also be free of chlorine, fluoride, metals, and certain minerals. That's why the really healthy raw kitchen relies on purified water. You can purify it yourself with filtration systems and distillation devices—I'll have more to say about that in chapter 7 on page 81. You can also have water delivered to your home. You can also buy distilled water—just add a pinch of evaporated sea salt to remineralize it.

If you buy your water, be wary of plastic bottles. Whether they are cloudy plastic or clear, plastic bottles can transfer chemicals into the water you drink and use preparing your food. Check around. Create a demand! In many places you'll find that supermarkets will sell purified water from a dispenser that fills the bottles you yourself bring. This may be a good option for you. Invest in some glass bottles that you can cap, seal, and keep in the refrigerator.

## other raw foods

In your local supermarket you are likely to find certain raw foods lined up on the shelves beside their cooked cousins. Take olive oil, for example. As a raw-food eater you want to look for specific words on the label. For olive oil, that word is *cold-pressed.* If your oil is cold-pressed and unadulterated you have raw olive oil. To get the best quality, look for extra-virgin olive oil. But not all extra-virgin oil is cold-pressed, so read the labels carefully.

Though they may not be (and most likely are not) organically produced, you can find many of the dry spices you want in the supermarket as well.

Your supermarket may stock other raw essentials too, but if they don't and won't bring it in upon request, it's time to shop elsewhere. Recently some produce stores have caught on to the fact that their clients include raw foodists who want raw nuts and beans, especially the lentils, almonds, and chickpeas (also known as garbanzos or garbanzo beans) that are used in so many recipes. As a result they may carry these dry foods. But remember, the essence of raw food is that it is uncooked. Make sure it says "raw" on the label. Just because it is dried doesn't mean it's raw and before you eat these foods, they'll need to be soaked or sprouted. But be careful to check and see that you are getting *raw* beans and lentils. How can you be sure?

In the United States, labeling laws require that you be informed about what is raw and what is not. Intended principally as a way to keep you from buying raw foods without warning (as though they might not be good for you), these requirements actually serve to help you find what you do want! Try to avoid foods that aren't labeled "raw."

# farmers' market

Next try a local farmers' market. Once a standard source for local produce, the farmers' market in America has evolved into all sorts of forms. In some places farmers' markets are actually distribution centers for bulk shipments of fresh produce at cut-rate prices. Other farmers' markets are a sort of gourmet, fresh-foods store. Still others have evolved into flea markets. Some are simply road-side stands next to farms. And in some locations they are just what they started out as—sites where a wide variety of fresh, seasonal, local farmer's produce (and sometimes other locally produced foods such as meats and sometimes raw cheeses) are sold. If you have one of these farmers' markets nearby, make it a habit to shop there. If you're used to the selection in your supermarket, your local farmers won't have everything you may want, but what they do have is bound to be fresh. The produce may not be organic, but it will be full of nutrients that foods shipped over long distances are likely to have lost. But try for organic. Best of all, it will be more tasty and more nutritious because it is bound to have been picked close to its full ripeness when flavors and nutrients are at their peak. You will definitely have to do additional produce shopping at the supermarket, but it's usually well worth picking up what you can at the local farmers' market. Just steer clear of the candies and baked goods!

# straight from the farm

Of course, if you're in an area where the farm isn't too far away, you shouldn't overlook buying from the local farmer directly. I know, how retro! Most Americans today have never been to a farm. But all around the country—and not just in the United States—there are farmers within a reasonable driving distance. And if you can find ones who use organic techniques, consider it part of your service to your community and the world to support them. While attending the 2002 Winter Olympics in Utah with my hockey-player boyfriend, I struck out to find raw milk. Right outside Park City there was a farmer who was happy to oblige.

Unfortunately, in many states the sale of raw food or transporting it across state lines for commercial purposes—to sell it—is against the law. That's why in most health-food stores you'll find organic milk, but only the pasteurized kind. The reasons for this are twofold: the fear that illness may occur if you drink unpasteurized milk and, more important, the powerful dairy lobby that controls the industry and determines who profits from it and where. But just because you can't buy it in stores doesn't mean it's not for sale.

Though you won't find billboards advertising them, you can buy local raw-dairy products in rural communities everywhere. There are no TV ads featuring models and actors pitching these products, but in Pennsylvania, barely a couple hours from where I live in New York City, there are Amish and Mennonite farmers who sell organic eggs and unpasteurized (and unhomogenized) milk, cream, and butter. In Ontario, Canada, a country I consider home, I go to the Mennonites when I can for my fresh raw-dairy products. Some even make and sell delicious raw cheeses. Most of these farms and others like them throughout America and Canada don't have separate shops but sell their products right out of the barn for a few hours, six days of the week. Unless you live in a neighboring town it may not be practical to go there every week. But don't forget that you can freeze milk, and eggs will last a bit in the fridge. Besides, the prospect of coming home with the essential ingredient in raw ice cream—fresh, raw, whole cream—alone could make the trip worth it! Get to know a local farmer.

# produce
## markets

Nowadays, you'll also find produce markets in many places. Unlike the farmers' market or roadside stand, most produce markets are places where you'll find just about anything that is grown or shipped in from around the world. I have been in produce markets where I couldn't identify half the items for sale, could barely pronounce their names, and, best of all, the proprietors were proud of the fact that they could get anything you wanted! Seek out these stores. Shop there. Talk to the people who run the place. Get to know them and let them know you're a regular customer. Tell them what your preferences are and what you wish they would carry. Sometimes they will agree to bring in items that you want on a special-order basis.

Thai coconuts are a good example. Not to be confused with the dark, hard-shelled coconuts, these soft white-skinned coconuts are always sweet and their meat is milky. They are the only coconuts I'll use. They make great shakes and pies. They are hard to come by in most supermarkets and not always available at many produce markets either. It's not difficult for stores to stock them, but the demand for them isn't great enough. But if you befriend the proprietor of the local produce market, he may agree to bring some every Tuesday, for example, and then you can buy them for the week. Become a regular customer. It's worth cultivating this sort of relationship and knowing you can get the incredible foods you want when you want them.

# health-food
## stores

If you are unable to get your raw-food staples at the supermarket or local produce store, you may have to pick them up at the health-food store. These days there are other options, but when I first started eating raw, health-food stores

were the first place to look for many foods because they could *only* be found there. Less than a decade ago most health-food stores were tiny, cluttered mom-and-pop operations. But recently, as the health-and-fitness industries have grown, health-food stores have grown up too. Most are still small, independent stores crowded with all sorts of products you probably have never heard of. But others have become large, airy, open spaces with attractively displayed items. Surprisingly, even the small stores seem to carry a huge variety of ingredients, including just about everything else you might want or need to prepare multi-course raw meals. On this list are raw apple cider vinegar, unpasteurized miso, Udo's Choice oil, sun-dried tomatoes, seaweed, spirulina, and psyllium husks, and shabunombu (or raw soy sauce), for example.

# food
# co-ops

In many communities food-conscious citizens have joined together and formed food co-ops. The way co-ops work is simple. Using the "there's power in numbers" principle, people gather together in order to buy foods that they want in bulk from sources they can trust. This can potentially lead to three practical results. First, co-op members can have access to foods they might not otherwise be able to get. Second, they get to set the standard for what they eat. Third, they get the food they want at considerable savings. Of course, the level of commitment on the part of the members, the number of those who join (which translates into buying power), and their particular interests will all play a part in whether and to what extent you might want to join a food co-op. But in any community with a well-educated market and concentrated demand, co-ops can be the best place to find what you want and to meet other people who might share your raw-food eating desires. Many co-ops specialize in certain kinds of food. There are organic food co-ops. There are produce-only co-ops. And the most successful ones can be as large as your local supermarket. Gone are the days of a few countercultural types fetching cases of surplus bananas and peaches from the back of a station wagon. Co-ops have truly come of age. In

more and more places, co-op shopping is even open to nonmembers. Look into your local co-op.

# raw-food
## specialty stores

For those of us who live in places like Los Angeles and New York, where the raw-food community can support its own cottage industry, there are raw-food specialty stores. If you're lucky enough to live near one of the major centers of raw foodism you'll want to seek out such a place. Typically they don't have a huge selection of foods, but what they do offer are those special raw treats that once you've tried them start to grow on you. I admit that I have my personal favorites. Live Live (212-505-5504; www.live-live.com) at 261 E. Tenth Street in New York, right next door to Quintessence Restaurant. The proprietor, Christopher Dobrowolski, not only has the answers to any questions I have about raw food and the raw-food scene, he also sells some of the best flaxseed crackers anywhere and teaches you how to make *great* nut milks. And at Jubb's Longevity, David Jubb makes delicious raw food desserts, drinks, burgers, and more. See resources, page 166.

# the
## internet

UPS and FedEx have been bringing me more and more of the items I want to eat in recent years, which I've ordered on the Internet. I've found that there are some products that are simply better bought online—or only available there—and delivered right to your door. The organic fourteen-grain cereal that I eat for breakfast with nut milk and raw honey is one example. So too are the olives from rawfood.com. They are delicious, and in my opinion it's hard to find any to compete with them on store shelves. I buy them by the case and stock my

pantry. Of all the companies on the Internet where you can buy raw food, not including produce, Nature's First Law offers the best selection. You can order their products through my Web site, www.carolalt.com.

# natural–food
## supermarkets

The best thing that has happened for raw foodists is the recent boom in natural-food supermarkets. Maybe you have never seen one—and if you haven't, you're missing something. Whole Foods Market and Wild Oats are the two largest chains and their business is booming. It seems they can't build stores fast enough. I have been shopping at the Whole Foods Market in Toronto and New York City for several years. These are not raw-food stores—they cater to all sorts of natural, organic, raw, high-quality food customers. As a result you really have to pay as close attention to what you are buying as you would at any other supermarket. The differences, however, can't be overstated. When you enter the produce section (yes, it's right where it is in your usual supermarket) the fruits, vegetables, and herbs are all labeled "conventional" or "organic." Very often there will be both, side by side: conventionally grown limes here and organically grown limes next to them. The selection of produce is simply amazing. Chances are they'll have just about everything on your shopping list. One-stop shopping—that's my kind of store.

When I say "one-stop shopping," I don't mean just produce. In addition to great produce and the items that raw foodists usually go to the health-food store for, these markets sometimes carry a selection of raw nut-butters and raw, sashimi-grade fish. They offer organic beef that is high grade and can be eaten raw as carpaccio or tartare. (Always tell the butcher you plan to eat it this way, so he gives you his best meat—same for fish.) They also have a great selection of raw cheeses from the United States and around the world, and the staff keeps a list of which ones are raw. You can ask to try them. Chances are any raw cheese you may want will be at Whole Foods Market. (You'll find many of them

in Wild Oats too, but in my experience Whole Foods Market generally has a better raw cheese selection.)

One of the other advantages of chain stores catering to a clientele that wants healthy food is that because they buy and sell in volume their prices are fair and competitive with conventional supermarkets. One of the most common objections people have to eating raw is that fresh foods aren't cheap. Yes, it's true that it is cheaper to eat dead food than living food. But to preserve your health, you can't afford *not* to eat living food.

Many people mistakenly believe they live in a fresh- and raw-food no-man's-land. You might be surprised to learn that there is a natural-food supermarket near you. Literally from Little Rock to Sacramento, from Omaha to Louisville, they are turning up everywhere. If you don't see one near you, check the Whole Foods Market and Wild Oats Web sites (www.wholefoods.com and www.wildoats.com) to find out if they have one planned for your area. If not, e-mail them to let them know you'd like one. They need to hear from you. Tell them you're trying to eat raw. Tell them Carol Alt sent you. And when they put one in your hometown, you'll be able to take credit for your small contribution toward feeding an overfed but still hungry nation. (And while you're at it, you might even ask Wild Oats to increase their selection of raw cheeses to rival Whole Foods Market.)

Remember, once you have established your sources for raw foods and raw products, it becomes easier and easier to eat raw.

# 7 gizmos, gadgets, toys, and treasures to equip the raw kitchen

Walk into my Lower Manhattan apartment kitchen and what do you see? You've got it—an ordinary kitchen! People are often surprised to discover that my raw-food kitchen looks just about like anyone else's. Well, almost—I have no toaster. And behind the cupboard doors there aren't very many pots and pans (though I do have some). With few exceptions, the things I use to prepare and store raw foods aren't much different from those in most other American homes. Preparing raw food doesn't involve a major investment in all new appliances.

My recommendation for setting up a raw kitchen is to begin with what you already have. I'll bet you have a refrigerator and freezer. On your countertop you probably already have a blender. You may own a grater. If you do, you're off to a good start. The fact is that you need fewer devices to eat raw than you do to cook. It won't be long before you decide to give your waffle iron to that friend who has always wanted one or put the equipment you no longer need into a storage closet.

# basic equipment
## for the raw kitchen

After eight years of eating without cooking, I've found there are a few indispensable everyday counter appliances I'd find it hard to live without. It's also true that the more you eat raw the more likely you are to want a few additional or better gizmos and gadgets. Let's start with the basics.

## a blender

It hardly takes any convincing to persuade most people of the merits of a good blender. As a child, my mother used one. Of course, back then no one in our Long Island home ever heard of a fruit smoothie. Milk shakes were the popular item of the day. Today, I wouldn't think of drinking a shake from a fast-food restaurant or even a thick, old-fashioned, hand-scooped shake from a soda fountain: too many fillers and additives. I can make even more delicious, completely raw ones in the blender at home and feed my body at the same time. My favorite blended drink is a smoothie made of all-raw green powder, kefir, yogurt, fruit, and nut milk. For me, it's almost the perfect food, since green powder gives the nutrition that satisfies hunger, kefir contains an intense dosage of beneficial bacteria, and nut milk contains protein for long-term energy. But on top of that, smoothies are delicious, fresh, and full of vitamins and minerals, and oh so easy to make. You can vary the ingredients, but the one thing you need every time is a blender. With your blender, raw soups are a snap too!

I even make breakfast in my blender. An avocado drink with raw milk and greens, for example, sounds terrible, and even I avoided it for several years until one day I walked in on Dr. Brantley sucking it down. Cornered! So I joined in. Now it's not a morning without a morning blend—and I don't mean coffee.

I also use my blender to make nut milks. It's too easy. (Check out the recipes on page 122–123.) It also makes a great sorbet. And how about a cold soup on a hot afternoon? I'm tired of gazpacho. I want variety. Speaking of variety, I can make any soup that I like into a "warm" meal too. You'd be surprised how warm 118 degrees is. So I miss out on nothing.

A blender's versatility and usefulness is directly proportional to how powerful it is and how variable the speed settings are. That's why investing in a good one is smart. At the same time, you don't want a machine that gets too hot and nearly cooks the food in it. You want a blender that is safe for food at any speed and doesn't leak. If you talk to people who know their way around a kitchen and who eat raw—and even those who don't—discussions about blenders usually turn to the Vita-Mix brand. It's the best blender I've found. I love my Vita-Mix. The company puts out several models, and unfortunately they're not cheap. The Vita-Mix 5000 retails for $399 and the Super 5000 sells for $479. But if you can afford it, these machines will not only do an amazing job of blending, they'll handle serious food processing and can chop all sorts of things. I use mine all the time.

Vita-Mix machines seem to last forever, and the company even allows you to trade up to a newer or more powerful model. Vita-Mix's reconditioned older machines sell for a fraction of the price of buying new. Decide what your needs are. If you're not going to be preparing much of your own food, you can start out with the blender you probably already have in your kitchen. But if you think it's time to invest in a serious kitchen appliance—one your non-raw houseguests will find a use for as well—give a Vita-Mix serious consideration. A Vita-Mix will also double as a juicer, and the machine comes with a tape that shows you how to make soups, ice cream, and more. You can find out more at www.vitamix.com.

## a coffee grinder

Sometimes a blender, even a great blender like the Vita-Mix, is just too big for a small chopping or grinding job. Maybe you have a handful of fresh pine nuts for pesto sauce, or you want to chop some raw Pecorino-Romano cheese for Caesar salad. Of course you can chop or grate by hand, but *uck!* I turn to my small electric coffee grinder for these sorts of chores. A coffee grinder is designed to turn tough, dry coffee beans into dust. To do that, its motor has to be strong. There are small food processors on the market specifically designed to do small grinding, dicing, and chopping jobs. Perhaps you already use one. If you decide to buy one of these instead of a coffee grinder, be sure it has enough horsepower to do the job.

Just a commonsense word of warning about using the coffee grinder: save it for foods that don't yield a lot of liquid, because typically only the lid is removable and you can't immerse the grinder in water or run it through the dishwasher—you'll have to wipe it clean.

## an instant-read thermometer

With this simple kitchen tool, you can heat up soups and sauces to a comfortably warm temperature without compromising the nutritional value of the vitamins and enzymes. Instant-read thermometers are inexpensive and widely available.

## water purifier and water distiller

Water is the essence of life. Our bodies are made up of 55–65 percent water, so it stands to reason that the better the quality of the water you put into your body, the better off you'll be. Without water nothing lives. With a depletion of as little as 2 percent of our normal bodily water content, we begin to feel fatigued and even get a warning headache. Water, and good water, is very important. While most of our tap water shouldn't kill us on the spot and is *supposedly* safe to drink, it still contains toxic metals and other harmful substances such as chlorine.

Chlorine, cheap and effective, is added to water to kill bacteria. It was also used as a nerve gas in World War II and has been clinically associated with everything from birth defects to cancers. Tap water also typically includes fluo-

ride, a by-product of aluminum smelting. Aluminum has been linked to Alzheimer's disease. Even distilled bottled water, the safest of all waters, is put into cloudy plastic bottles that are thought to leech chemicals into the freshly distilled water they carry. When are the water companies going to get smarter? Consumers certainly are.

Some time ago I added a filtration system to my tap. I also recently bought a distiller that sits on the countertop and looks sort of like a coffeemaker to replace the distilled, purified, bottled water I seemed to buy by the truckload. It's a Waterwise Model 8800, and I couldn't be happier with it. I take purified tap water and run a gallon at a time through the distiller. In four hours it's ready. Then I put the purified water in the fridge to use for all my drinking and food preparation. (See the Resources section for more information on companies like Custom Air & Water.)

## a spiralizer

If there has ever been an appliance that to me was worth every cent you spend on it, this one is it! Sold for under $30, the Spiral Slicer (formerly sold as Saladacco) is the ultimate raw kitchen bargain. What makes this hand-operated device so special is that it cuts vegetables into shapes. Originally designed to make cute, decorative garnishes, it transforms vegetables such as carrots, cucumbers, sweet potatoes, and radishes into thin slices, julienne strips, cubes, or fine strands. This gadget is great for making salads and cole slaw, of course, but in my opinion best of all is that you can make raw "pasta." Run a butternut squash or zucchini through the spiralizer, and out comes a raw version of angel hair pasta—without the cooked wheat gluten—that you will love. (Check out the Spaghetti al Pesto on page 150.)

## a vacuum storage system

There was a time in human history not so long ago when food was caught, harvested, and prepared fresh each day. Forget that! It didn't take long for humans to get smart about preserving and storing food so we could eat it when we wanted it, not just when we could find it or when it was in season.

These days we buy food and just pop it into the fridge. All in all, refrigeration is a good food-preservation choice. It's easy, and quick, and lowering the ambi-

ent temperature holds the growth of bacteria and other microorganisms in check, retarding spoiling.

But eventually all food goes bad in the fridge. What is the single most important factor in the transformation? Air. Enveloped in the air that is all around it, the chemical composition of food immediately begins to change and it changes very quickly, even before you can actually see it. Before visible decay sets in, foods start losing potency as a life source. What was a living food, full of essential enzymes, is in the process of dying. What is dying starts decaying. But even before it begins to noticeably decay it is losing its ability to nourish you.

Every refrigerator circulates air. Inside even "airtight" plastic refrigerator storage containers there is a sealed-in pocket of air. It may not be *fresh* air but it is still air. The oxygen in air is what predatory microorganisms need to grow and overtake a food source, whether it is raw or not. So unless you eat foods right when you prepare them and then throw away any leftovers, you have to find a way to keep your food from the air to capture your food's freshness, preserve its raw nutrients a little longer, and slow down the process of spoiling and decay. The answer? Vacuum storage.

Most of the foods in my fridge are vacuum sealed. I use a vacuum system called VacSy, put out by Zepter International. (There are others on the market, ones that are sold on QVC for example, but I've never had a problem with my Zepter.) At first glance, the containers in my fridge look pretty much like the two-piece container-and-lid Tupperware types many of us grew up with. They also come in all shapes and sizes. But looks can be deceiving. Here's how they differ: First, because they are made of glass, the containers don't absorb any of the food or discolor; they also have durable polycarbonate lids, and silicone seals. Second, each lid has a valve in the center. Once you put your food in the container and put on the lid, you'll notice it doesn't snap on. You insert a hand-held vacuum pump, smaller than a curling iron, into the valve, the lid sucks on and clamps down. Then you lock it. That's it! It's so simple. The containers and lids are dishwasher safe and because they are made from glass they don't warp or discolor over time. They're clear, so with just a glance you can see exactly what it is you have in the fridge. Most important, they keep food from spoiling as quickly as it would in old-fashioned containers you probably use now.

When I lived in LA, I shopped at the Santa Monica Farmers' Market. One day I came home with lots of fresh organic food. Then I got a call—on short notice I needed to be in Europe. None of my neighbors were home so I couldn't give my fresh produce away, and I was not about to toss all the fruits and vegetables I just bought. I figured this would be the perfect Zepter test. I packed all my lettuce and veggies into the containers (cheeses too, no meat or fish), and left town. I ended up coming home some time later, forgetting at this point that I had left fresh food in the fridge. I got home hungry and started scrounging. I opened the refrigerator and to my happy surprise there was my produce, all looking in good form. The taste test was next, and pretty much everything passed with flying colors. I mean, lettuce usually lasts—what—about a week at most?

A basic Zepter outfit with four storage containers and lids, a cap for sealing bottles, and the vacuum pump runs about $200. Of course, you can buy additional pieces. Zepter products are very popular in Europe but are not easy to find in stores in the United States. Like the Vita-Mix, you can get them online.

The second sort of vacuum system uses plastic bags—sort of like a Ziploc but without the air. I bought one for my boyfriend so he could freeze his stash of organic meats. QVC offers a good one on TV. It's convenient and the bags don't take up much space.

One last word: if there is any indication that foods are going bad, *throw* them out. Raw meats are best eaten the day they are made, vacuum-sealed and stored for a day, or frozen (freezing doesn't necessarily destroy enzymes).

# optional additions
## to the raw kitchen

I'll bet somewhere in the back of every woman's mind is a dream kitchen full of optional additions. If I close my eyes and imagine the raw-food kitchen of my dreams, there are a few items that make the picture complete (besides a full-time chef!).

## a dehydrator

In some hot climates, you can dry foods in the sun, but the most efficient method, however, is to use a dehydrator. Dehydrators aren't too expensive, with retail prices in the range of $100 to $200. A company called Excalibur makes 5-tray and 9-tray dehydrators that are popular with raw foodists.

Why is a dehydrator so helpful? Much of conventional food preparation depends on baking to evaporate and to set liquids and semisolids like cake batter or bread dough. But the temperatures required are high, much too high for anything to remain raw. Using a dehydrator, the temperatures are low but the effect is much the same. Dehydrating—taking the water out—can transform a brown batter into delicious carob cake or a seedy mush into crisp flaxseed crackers. And then there are the tasty nut snacks, dried fruits, and other delicious snacks and ingredients.

## a sprouter

You really don't need a sprouter to make your own sprouts. When I'm home, I sprout the traditional way—I buy them in the store. All kidding aside, using a jar, cheesecloth, and water works just as well. I confess I *have* sprouted and germinated nuts, grains, and seeds this way on occasion. (Actually, I use a new stocking rather than cheesecloth to keep bugs out of the jar). It's simple and hardly any work; see page 163 for instructions. Many people who own them swear by their sprouters.

## a juicer

Okay, I myself don't actually own a juicer. I talked my boyfriend into making that investment! When I'm in Manhattan, however, where juice bars are easier to find than parking spots, I usually let someone else blend my heartier organic vegetable juices, and I use my blender to make simple green drinks at home. For me this makes sense because a really good vegetable blend means getting the right fresh organic ingredients and making and drinking the juice right away. Since I travel a lot, going out to buy the ingredients I need to make myself some juice, and buying just the right amounts so they are fresh, is more effort than just stopping in at a juice bar where all day long they do just one

thing: extract juice from pulp and serve it up. It's no muss, no fuss, nothing to clean up. No shopping for just the right combination of carrots, celery, wheat-grass, parsley, spinach, kale, ginger, sprouts, and cucumbers. It's fast food gone raw and healthy! You can vacuum-seal juices. They sometimes last up to three days.

As I mention in the section on blenders, certain high-end blenders can double as juicers. But a complete raw kitchen—more complete than mine—would ultimately have a full-fledged, heavy-duty juicer in it.

This piece of equipment definitely isn't like Grandma's old orange squeezer—making a vegetable juice really can't be done by hand without hard work and a lot of waste. Besides, in the time it would take to hand-juice the ingredients much of its nutrition would be lost through contact with oxygen in the air. The best juicers use a very efficient, dual-gear extraction method instead of the "centrifugal mastication" extraction process used by blenders. The typical home blender that chops and spins may release only one-quarter of the enzymes a dual-gear juicer does. What you get from a blender is fresh and raw but not nearly as potent.

When it comes to buying a juicer the old adage is true: you get what you pay for. Then again, unless you have a family of five or intend to use your juicer for half a lifetime, chances are you don't need a top-of-the-line machine. Still it's worth getting a good juicer that will turn those veggies into juice without making scary grinding sounds and smelling of burning rubber while wasting your fresh produce. If you buy one, get a reliable model. Here are some of the ones that some raw foodists prefer.

The top-of-the-line in-home juicer may be the Samson Ultra Twin Gear (Kempo) Juicer. It is quiet, efficient, and not only separates juices from veggie pulp but makes clear fruit juices and sorbets. It even has an attachment to turn out vegetable pasta and noodles. Its ten-year warranty is a small offset to the $499 retail price, but if you shop around you may be able to find a substantial discount. Those who don't rate the Samson "tops" usually prefer the Green Power Gold Juice Extractor, whose makers boast of its high power but slow grinding and compression speed. It seems that when vegetables are ground slowly and compressed, toxic metals with high specific gravities such as mercury

and lead naturally bind with the cellulose (pulp) that is discarded. It retails for more than the Sampson—$650—but if you keep a lookout you should find a deep discount. I've seen it for just over $400. It comes with a two-year warranty.

An additional benefit from these two machines is that they both juice wheat-grass. Notoriously hard to extract, many raw foodists use a slow-turning, manual juicer such as the Stainless Steel Wheatgrass Juicer by Back to Basics ($119 retail) to handle this nutritionally superpotent food. There are also a number of motorized juicers on the market designed specifically for wheatgrass. (I just buy E3live, a flash-frozen green supplement that's just as good as wheat grass.)

Besides the highly efficient dual-gear juicers, there's a wide array of masticating, centrifugal, centrifugal-ejection, and single-auger juicers of varying quality that are designed for home use, with prices ranging from $100 to $250.

# 8

# eating out

## and raw entertaining: where, when, how, and with whom to dine

You can't stick to a hectic schedule and lead a professional life and only eat at raw restaurants. There are too few of them. Besides, if you ate only with other raw foodists you'd be dining alone five nights a week. ✳ In this chapter I'd like to show you how you can eat raw and still have a social life like anyone else. That may mean eating at places that are not necessarily known for their raw-food menu. It includes sharing raw food with your friends and family on your own turf. And if you have a raw restaurant nearby, I'd like to help make it easy for you

to take people there, to introduce them to the joys and pleasures of eating raw and maybe ease them into a healthier, raw-food lifestyle.

I can already imagine your question: if I eat only raw food—except, of course, for the occasional guilty cooked food—how can I possibly go out and have dinner with friends who eat everything cooked?

Let me assure you that you won't need to make everyone else feel uncomfortable over your eating raw. It's true, when word gets around some people you know and cherish may whisper, "Maybe we shouldn't invite Carol because I hear she doesn't eat cooked food anymore." Just remember, they're not trying to snub you. I think their real intention is to show respect. So don't take it personally if you find yourself somehow overlooked for a dinner invitation. What's most important is for you to know that there's no need to let raw food curtail your relationships and activities. And the quicker you learn how to eat raw wherever you are, the sooner your friends will be surprised at how easy it is for you to blend in now the same way you always did before. Once again you'll be invited everywhere.

# restaurants

For the raw foodist, much like trying to do your grocery shopping at the local neighborhood supermarket, going out to eat at a typical restaurant is less than ideal—but it can be easier than you might think. If it's up to me and I'm asked where I'd like to go for lunch or dinner, of course I choose a place that has lots of raw options nestled among the cooked ones my friends are sure to want. Japanese is usually easy because sashimi—the raw fish used in making varieties of sushi—is there on the menu along with salads and vegetables that can be served raw. My New York restaurants of choice are Nobu and Sushi Samba because they serve marinated fish and ceviches. I also love to eat at Morton's Steak House. Yes, a steak house is at the top of my list of places to eat raw. The reason is simple. Morton's makes delicious fish and meats that I am able to eat seared as well as a wide variety of greens and salads. And, of course, a steakhouse menu has something for just about anyone else I may be dining with. (Check with your local steak house to find out where they get their meat and if they feel it's safe to serve seared.)

If you're not the one choosing where to eat, try to find out in advance where you'll be going. If it's a place that's popular and they have a lot of turnover there is a much better chance that their food is fresh and less likely to be on the edge of spoiling. I have found that as long as the food a restaurant serves is fresh, I can eat a meal almost anywhere. And sometimes I'm very pleasantly surprised at what I find. For example, I went to a Greek restaurant recently that didn't serve any raw fish, but they had such fresh fish the owner was comfortable enough to make me the most delicious swordfish carpaccio and he rounded up a bunch of greens and garnishes for the best, most unusual salad. Actually, I had two or three orders of the carpaccio. As someone who eats raw, you may only be able to eat two or three of the items listed on the menu. But the good news is that you can have as much of it as you want!

If I have the chance, I like to call ahead and ask the chef or the maître d' some questions. Try to make yourself do this. Begin by letting them know that you eat raw (but don't be surprised if they make the same assumptions that so many other people do, for example, that raw foodists only eat salads). Tell them what sorts of things you like to eat. I'm fond of sea bass and swordfish if they are only slightly grilled outside, leaving the inside warm but still raw. I usually mention this. Then ask them what's on their menu. Ask if they would have a problem making certain items seared—the "fresh fish of the day," for example. If they hesitate and don't have a suggestion for something that they could prepare and serve raw, it's reasonable to assume that their food isn't safe for you to eat, whether it's raw or not. When that happens to me, I plan on just ordering a salad and fruit. I don't risk food poisoning. I have never, not once, gotten sick from eating raw food in a restaurant and I don't care to. I'm not one to take chances.

I have been known to show up at a restaurant and say, "I want a salad made from everything that you have that is raw in your kitchen." Even the most raw-food-unfriendly establishment probably can be coaxed to cut up one piece of each variety of fresh vegetable they have. At a bare minimum that usually means celery, peppers, tomatoes, carrots, romaine and some other sort of lettuce, onions if you want them, and perhaps even mesclun greens and avocados. It often includes more. A salad may not be the sort of gourmet culinary delight that you were hoping for, but for just one meal out it will at least fill you up, especially if you can follow it up with fresh fruit for dessert.

Of course, if I know before going out to eat that the raw menu choices will be few or possibly only a salad, I have something to eat before I head out the door. Carol's Rule Number 1 for Eating Out: don't ever leave home if you are starving!

If you go out hungry you're likely to devour the first thing that comes to the table—the bread! I've already told the story about how I suffered from sinus and colds I now know were directly tied to eating bread and other wheat-gluten products. Though I didn't know it at the time, for many years bread was making me sick, as I believe it does so to many other people. Like most people I had no idea there was any connection between my various interrelated illnesses—colds, sinus problems, flu, headaches—and my deadly, daily bread and pasta products intake. Many people find that cooked or baked wheat gluten acts like sugar in one's system and is a toxin to the body. Knowing that, the last thing you need to do is to sit down at the table in a restaurant and begin nibbling on the bread because you're hungry and it's your first and only immediate option. I typically have a piece of raw cheese, maybe some guacamole, and a couple of raw flaxseed crackers (available online at carolalt.com) or maybe a piece of sprouted "fruit and nut" Manna Bread to take the edge off my hunger before leaving home. I never touch the bread at a restaurant.

Rule Number 2: if you're going to dinner straight from the office, bring raw-milk cheese or germinated almonds with you when you go to work because they make a good snack anytime and are easy keep on hand. I know this rule sounds kind of quirky, but it's not. Just a little bit of these two raw sources of fats and proteins seem to suppress hunger while providing you the nutrients you need to make it through even the most Spartan of raw menus.

I also never take my own food with me to a restaurant. I know some people on special diets do this, but eating raw isn't a special diet; it's a lifestyle. I try to adapt wherever I go and I don't wish to make my dinner companions uncomfortable or insult the restaurant staff by showing up with my own ice chest full of food. I have been known to take along certain spices, however. I typically carry along some Celtic sea salt in a small shaker. I also often travel with a small squeeze bottle of cold-pressed olive oil and raw apple cider vinegar dressing. Fill up the bottle at home and then put it in your (or your wife's) purse and go. It's easy.

Of course, if you're inviting people to eat with you, out or at home, the decisions about what will be served rest in your hands. As long as you're sensitive to your colleagues, friends, and family members you should have no problems. In fact, you may find that they are curious about raw food and want to try out new dishes with you that they wouldn't on their own. Remember, take it easy. (They might also want to hear how your health improved after a couple months of eating raw.)

# picnics

One good meal choice for raw foodists is a picnic. The reason is simple. Many of the raw-food dishes that non-raw foodists immediately seem to like are natural picnic selections. There are so many varieties of raw cheeses available, made from cow's, goat's, and sheep's milk, that putting together a cheese plate is easy. When you're shopping at the local Whole Foods Market or Wild Oats or the cheese shop, just remember to ask for the raw-milk varieties. There are all sorts of salads that are perfect for a picnic. Just among the recipes in this book they run the gamut from a lentil salad (page 135) to a red and green cabbage cole slaw (page 136) and a broccoli salad (page 133) that I picked up from my friend Marybeth. With salads, the possibilities are endless. And don't forget dipping favorites such as raw hummus, guacamole, and salsa. Even though raw chips and crackers are certain to stand out as new and different your guests are likely to enjoy them.

Nothing in your picnic basket should send up red flags as being 100 percent raw. Don't be surprised, however, if you hear people around you saying with delight, "this food all tastes so fresh!" You can tell them with pride that it tastes fresh because it *is* fresh and very few of us are accustomed to routinely eating truly fresh foods.

Just as I do for a picnic, I often pack food to take with me in the car when I'm going on a trip. There's no reason for me to stop for cooked junk food if I have something good to eat with me. Remember to pack raw foods in airtight containers and not to leave them out of refrigeration for too long.

# raw
## restaurants

I've become more and more inclined to take people to raw restaurants because I've gotten such good feedback about the food. That way, they can experience the foods I love and that have become such a part of my life. Even though I can't imagine those I know and love continuing to eat cooked food day in and day out, I'm not the heavy-handed "convert the unrepentant dead-food eater" type. I prefer a gentler, subtler approach. I know that anyone who walks through the door of a raw-food restaurant like Quintessence or Pure Food & Wine and sits down and eats a meal with me is going to walk out glad that they did. I have yet to leave with someone who was disappointed. Not everyone is equally excited, but no one walks away with regrets—the food is just so good. And many people are positively shocked because they couldn't begin to imagine how delicious and diverse well-prepared raw food really is.

If you have never been in a raw restaurant before, or if you have and want some hints on how to introduce others to eating raw, I'll share with you a few simple steps.

The first thing I do, after getting seated and inevitably talking about the particular place, is to ask my guests to read the menu. This is important because people tend to have a lot of misconceptions about eating raw, and seeing what they may eat in black and white makes it apparent that what awaits them is not so foreign at all. There are certain ingredients that may seem new or unusual, but all in all the menu reads like any other menu. Of course, just because something raw has the same name as something cooked doesn't make it the same. But overall, reading a raw-food menu is nothing like the puzzling experience you may have had the first time you sat down in an Indian or a Thai restaurant.

Once my guests have had a chance to look over the menu and I mention some of my favorite dishes, I explain to them about the food not being hot (and I don't mean spicy). But hot is a relative term. So what is hot? For the sake of raw food the cutoff temperature is when foods begin chemically and structurally to be altered, more or less 118 degrees F. As a result, not all raw soups are served refrigerated, and "pastas" are definitely not served steaming.

I'm inclined to suggest something from the menu that is close to what they already know. Pesto pasta is a good example. The texture is similar to that of angel hair pasta served al dente and the sauce is made from pine nuts, olive oil, basil, and garlic—the same essential ingredients in the cooked pesto sauces they have had before. Though it is served at room temperature there is no mistaking the fact that the textures and flavors are familiar ones, so this is indeed "pesto pasta."

Usually I order several entrées to share with my guests so that they can try a little of each and decide (and eat more of) what they personally prefer. All food, raw or cooked, is alike in this way: we each have our individual favorite dishes and everyone's are different. Don't feel you need to like everything. As with cooked food it's perfectly okay not to like every dish you try. This is true of raw restaurants as well. If you ask those of us in New York City who have access to more than one raw restaurant, you will hear the names of several different favorite places to eat, like "Counter," "Pure Food & Wine," or "Caravan of Dreams." We all have different tastes. You may think the food at my favorite place is too spicy and I may find your favorite's too bland. People may prefer this dish here and that dish there. Others like them the other way around. Don't expect everyone to love everything just as you do.

Over time, as we try new things, our palates change. As you eat more and more raw foods you will begin to grow used to certain tastes that seemed foreign not so long before. Some of these you'll grow to love and crave. You may even begin to wonder how it was you could have "missed out" for so many years. What initially seem to be unusual tastes or textures become familiar everyday ones. Other tastes and textures, those of cooked foods in particular, will begin to seem unusual and possibly even unappealing to you over time.

Chain restaurants, fast-food joints, and even local diners like the ones that I grew up with on Long Island dot the map all over North America. That's a lot of cooked food everywhere you turn. I remember when I was working in Italy in the mid-1980s and Rome's first fast-food restaurant opened right in the shadow of the Spanish Steps. The Italians were torn between tradition and the unpleasant wave of the future—the rush for the unhealthy but quick and easy "Dollar Menu." Since then, fast-food restaurants have spread all over that country and now there is hardly a place in the world where they aren't known.

At the same time, because eating out at restaurants is more common and popular than it ever was before and so is raw food, there are more and more raw-food restaurants cropping up all the time. No, I doubt there's a wave of raw fast-food chains on the horizon. But it's only a matter of time before conventional cooked-food restaurants begin to feature specifically planned raw menu items—more than the often not-too-healthy salad selections with *cooked* dressings and croutons. And, as with fresh-food markets like Whole Foods and Wild Oats, I predict that very soon you'll see all-raw restaurants beginning to sprout up all over the land. Meanwhile, you owe it to yourself to seek out any raw restaurants near you and taste some of the amazingly delicious raw culinary possibilities. And if you visit a new city, seek out these restaurants. Especially if you live somewhere without a raw-food restaurant.

# q&a

## my answers to those who are hesitant, scared, apprehensive, or simply uncertain

I'm inquisitive by nature. I like to learn things. I like to figure things out. So I ask lots of questions. While writing this book, I've become more aware of aspects of eating raw that, despite eight years as a raw foodist, I either knew little about or simply took for granted. So, as usual, I've asked questions and am sharing the answers I found here in this book. Before starting any lifestyle change, everyone should ask questions, seek answers from different sources (I've found the Internet is a good place to cross-reference), including any doctors you know.

People also come up to me to ask me about the raw-food lifestyle. I like answering their questions the best way I can with the information I've gathered from doctors and other raw foodists. If you're anything like me (or them) you have your own questions about eating raw.

As you read this you may be standing in a bookstore just browsing *Eating in the Raw*. Or maybe you bought the book, took it home, and had just begun to look at it when you stopped at this chapter because you wanted some quick answers. Or perhaps you've read every page of the book up to this point but you still have some doubts or uncertainties or you just need a nudge to get going. It's a big step that you want to take, but you need more reassurance that it's the right thing for you to do. (It helps if you check with your doctor first, as always.)

If you're any one of these people this chapter is for you. Here are some of the most frequently asked questions people have asked me about raw food—and the answers you may need.

## how do i know if something is raw?

"We won't be fooled again," is how the old Who song goes. Look for the word *raw* on the label. In the United States raw foods must say they are raw. They can also say *cold-pressed* (in the case of oils), *unpasteurized* (for dairy products), and *sprouted* (if it's a product made from grains). Some foods may be labeled with the words *cru, crude,* or *unprocessed.* Read the label, and look at every ingredient. Here the manufacturer legally shouldn't be able to mislead.

And I do mean mislead. Plenty of food companies seem to be jumping on the raw bandwagon and they want to reap the "pro-seeds" without sowing the seeds first. For example, I bought some sprouted bread the other day. The label on the front boasted "sprouted" in large letters, so I didn't bother reading the ingredients on the back. When I got it home and opened the bread I immediately noticed that it looked like any other bread you'd buy off the shelf. I mean it looked like plain ol' white bread. So I started to read the ingredients and what did I find? The first ingredient was sprouted but next was white flour, followed by all the regular cooked ingredients. Now I stick with Ezekiel or Genesis bread.

Don't be fooled by foods like store-bought hummus that are in the refriger-

ated section and served up cold. Just because it's cold doesn't make it raw. All the ingredients are cooked. There's usually not one drop of raw oil or one uncooked chickpea in the hummus you usually buy.

If you have to ask if something is raw, you can almost be certain it isn't. Most people who work in a supermarket or restaurant never think about whether something is raw or not. And they're not likely to know much about ingredients either. It's not a criticism, just a recognition that they don't think along such lines.

## how hard is it to eat this way?

For me, it was the easiest thing I ever did because I immediately saw the benefits. There's no doubt that it's easier for most people to eat anything they feel like, anywhere, anytime. But I don't recommend it. I told you what the consequences were for me. I experienced headaches, acid indigestion, sinus problems, weight gain, PMS, bloating, and degenerative disease that completely changed for me by cutting out cooked food.

For me it was a lot healthier, and in a way, easier, to eat anything I wanted in moderation, but *raw*. So that's what I do. The difference in how your body processes raw food is explained in chapter 3. In what to me is no doubt some God-given, natural plan, if we eat unprocessed, raw foods, and the right supplements (see your doctor for the best supplements and raw foods for you), our bodies seem to regulate themselves. Our bodies seem to know when to stop eating. It doesn't eat and then hunger for more and more and more. It feels satisfied when it *is* satisfied.

Also, once you begin to think about food differently and to see raw food as food and cooked food as garbage (often tasty garbage, no doubt), it becomes pretty easy to eat it raw. Practically speaking, it's all a matter of changing habits. Because we have so little experience of eating really delicious raw food, we tend to think that living on food that hasn't been cooked should be hard. But raw food is delicious—and especially when you taste recipes that are simply incredible—you'll find as I did that it's not hard to "eat this way" at all. Once you get used to raw food's pleasures and benefits I believe you'll find it hard *not* to choose raw over cooked food.

One of my reasons for writing this book is to make eating raw easy, whether you're shopping for food, preparing it, having guests over, or going out to eat. If you haven't read the rest of the book, read it. I think you'll become convinced that it's not hard at all.

## but aren't you hungry? like all models you're very thin.

Don't confuse being trim with being hungry. When I was eating cooked food and starving myself to stay thin as a model, I was very literally hungry almost all of the time. I am never hungry now. I eat all the time. I feel great. I have lots of energy. I'm thin now, but I'm not hungry at all.

## what do you mean, "eat all you want"?

Well, before I started to eat raw, I deprived myself of many of the things I liked to eat: desserts, snacks like cookies, and especially cheeses. Now that I'm eating raw, I've added back raw cheeses (just never a mountain of any one type, since the body seems to thrive on variety). And since I've found raw-food stores, restaurants, and Internet sites that have raw pies, cookies, snacks, and other specialties that satisfy my cravings for these types of foods, I have even added these back into my diet too!

And raw food is just so satisfying. Now, I find that even if I want to eat two pieces of raw coconut cream pie after a raw dinner, I usually can't fit it in. I usually can't finish one piece for that matter! I'm just so satisfied!

Just the other night, I took a new friend of mine, Dan, to Quintessence restaurant to eat. Dan's remarks seemed to sum up the raw-food experience; "You know," he said, "I came here so hungry and thought that I would want to eat a ton of food. I wanted to order everything on the menu. But after this normal-sized meal, I don't feel a heavy, weighed-down full—I feel a satisfied full. And everything tasted so . . . fresh. I feel life behind my eyes. Strange."

Why should this be strange? Shouldn't food revive us and give us vitality and life? As Dan Hoyt explained to us, most raw foods are nutrient-dense foods. So they satisfy your body and you stop eating before your stomach is too full!

## when i hear "raw" somehow i think "vegetarian," but it doesn't sound as though you're talking about being a vegetarian. are you?

It's not surprising that you should be confused. Most of the people who are best known as raw foodists are also vegetarians or vegans. I'm not. The two people who have most influenced me over the years are Timothy Brantley, ND, an independent researcher in Southern California, and more recently Nicholas Gonzalez, MD, a physician in New York City. When I set out to find the most competent professionals I could to help me, I didn't go looking for "meat-eating raw foodists." I just wanted the best help I could find. I don't think Drs. Brantley and Gonzalez have ever met one another. But both believe that for most of us there are good reasons to eat more than just vegetable matter.

I'm not at odds with those who, for a variety of reasons, are opposed to eating animal products. Most of my raw-foodist friends are either vegetarians or vegans of one sort or another. It's clear to me that whether you do or do not eat meat, fish, dairy, even honey (which some strict vegans will not), eating fresh raw food is better for you than, for example, eating a cooked vegetarian diet. For more on the distinctions among vegan, vegetarian, and related other terms, take a look at chapter 4. To understand more about meat eating, vegetable eating, why eating raw is better for you than any cooked diet, and why I eat the way I do, read chapter 3, which Dr. Gonzalez contributed to.

## it sounds as though you don't really care about fat in your diet. isn't it important to watch your fat intake?

I care tremendously about fat in my diet and in fact to me the more I get the better! But for me, it absolutely, positively *must* be raw or I won't eat it even if I'm starving. The best oils I've found are raw coconut, olive, Udo's Choice, and Premier Research Labs EFA oils.

According to Dr. Gonzalez, carbohydrates are a minor component of body structure compared to proteins and fats. If a body cannot molecularly read a cooked fat, it is then more easily *stored* then metabolized. Therefore the body, which needs essential fatty acids (omega 9 and omega 3 and only a moderate

amount of omega 6) from fats for things like the immune system, begins to break down. No wonder there is so much disease and sickness: we live in a no-fat/low-fat/cooked-fat society.

More important to me, my skin changed for the better with the increase in raw oils, and believe it or not according to Robert Marshall PhD CCN old fats are chased out of your system through a preferential exchange with the healthy fats found in raw foods.

## i've heard that eating raw is dangerous. be honest. isn't it?

To be honest, I have not had any problems myself. But eating raw food is not like eating it cooked. As you know, all raw food is more perishable than cooked food, so you really need to get it fresh—that means knowing your food sources, and your sources' sources. You should always try to get your foods organic too—especially if you are eating them raw.

Most raw foodists I know are vegan, so they eat no animal products. This is, of course, safer in terms of bacteria because they make most of their dishes out of nuts, fruits, and vegetables. And most people know how long fruits and vegetables last. Most of the recipes I have included in this book are based on fresh produce and raw-milk cheese. When you feel comfortable enough to eat fish and meat raw, then go ahead and do so, but be certain of the freshness of your food.

Seek out reputable restaurants that serve tartars, sashimi, ceviches, and other raw animal products. Always make sure of high turnover and get recommendations from friends and family. If you are eating something raw, make sure the proprietor knows this and is comfortable with serving raw food. Sometimes, I opt to be extra-safe by eating only salad for dinner and then fruit for dessert.

Cheese and other dairy products should come from licensed cheese vendors. You should ask the vendor how long the cheese will last and how long it's been since it was made.

I have had great success with raw foods. They changed my life. But the most important thing to remember is to partner with a doctor or nutritionist who can give you in-depth advice on balancing your raw diet and finding the supplements that are right for you. Always be curious, sensible, and educated.

But let's face it—there are a lot of people who have a lot invested in cooked

food. I mean *a lot of people!* Some doctors, nutritionists, not to mention those in the restaurant business and the food industry, have a stake in cooked food. It's cheaper and keeps longer and there is a culture of disbelief about the benefits of eating raw among people whose livelihood is tied to cooked food—either selling it, making it, or supposedly (and indeed sometimes actually) curing people who suffer the consequences of it—and they are not likely to walk away from it. So of course if they can scare you away from eating raw by telling you "it's dangerous," it's to their advantage. Their livelihood is at stake. So be sure to seek out medical advice from people who understand the raw-food point of view.

## what about bacteria and things like salmonella in eggs? surely there must be a reason the government makes sure milk is pasteurized.

In the nineteenth century when Louis Pasteur developed the process of pasteurization, his technique amounted to a revolution in preserving foods. It's very simple. By raising the temperature of milk, for example, to a level where natural bacteria die but the milk does not actually boil (milk boils at 214°F.—pasteurization is at 165°F.), it's possible to slow down the natural process of spoilage and give the milk a longer shelf life. But are the natural bacteria always unhealthy? Here's where people get confused.

What I've found is bacteria in themselves are not bad. We all have bacteria living in us all the time and we ingest some bacteria that are essentially harmless. What does us harm are certain strains of microorganisms that our bodies are not accustomed to as well as foods that are no longer living but "spoiled."

One way to minimize and even effectively eliminate the chance of that happening is to eliminate the bacteria entirely. The trade-off is that in doing so, by pasteurizing or cooking, we also eliminate the essential, living substances— the enzymes and proteins—that are essential for us to be healthy over the long term, making us less immune and weaker. At the same time we become less resistant to the effects of bacteria we might inadvertently ingest or inhale.

Ironically, the process developed by Pasteur nearly a century and a half ago is in my opinion no longer necessary. The more recent developments of wide-

spread refrigeration and inexpensive and effective vacuum sealing can hold back spoilage without altering a food's structure. But pasteurization is quick and effective, and so it continues. Those who manufacture, pack, ship, and sell food can count on it. It's cheap and that keeps food prices down too. The practices of routine pasteurization along with cooking have done something else to our supply of food. They have allowed food producers to be careless with the food they produce and allow longer shipping time because these cooked foods with preservatives don't spoil.

## what do you miss most about eating cooked food?

Honestly, I really don't miss it. I like my popcorn. It's kind of hard to have popcorn that is uncooked. With few exceptions, however, anything you eat cooked has a raw equivalent. I am eating a greater variety of foods now than I was when I was eating cooked foods. And now I even eat food I forbade myself to eat before I ate raw, like my beloved cheeses. Everything I'm eating now tastes so good and is so good for me that it's hard to miss what I now think once made me sick, always left me hungry for more, and never really satisfied me—cooked food.

## my great-uncle lived to be 105 and smoked Camel unfilters—so why would I have to watch my health if the members of my family tend to live long?

Dr. Timothy Brantley once told me, "It is not about the length of life—I mean, I could get hit by a bus stepping off the curb—it is about the quality of life." Eating raw food helped me to eliminate the everyday illnesses that destroyed my quality of life.

And even though occasionally someone with unhealthy habits lives a very long life, it's the exception rather than the rule. Today in America, one in three people dies of cancer, and one in two dies of heart disease. What are we doing differently now than we did even 100 years ago? We are infusing our food and our environment with chemicals. Hormones, insecticides, irradiation, preservatives . . . these are just some of the things that come to mind.

A couple of generations ago, people grew up eating dairy products that were usually *unpasteurized.* Most animals weren't injected with hormones and crops were rotated and fed without the use of chemical pesticides. After the 1950s, surplus World War II chemicals were converted into agricultural products and soils became contaminated and depleted. Genetic alteration affected the nature of the crops we eat. I think these more recent events have a great effect on our food supply, and thus our health as a whole.

## i'm not convinced i can go totally raw right now. what sorts of things can i do immediately to begin reaping the benefits of eating raw food?

There's no need to go totally raw right away. Here are just a few helpful hints to get you started:

⁜ When cooking, add cold-pressed olive oil *afterward.* If you're making a pasta sauce, for example, don't use oil at all with your tomatoes to get the sauce started. Stew them in water and then, just before you're ready to serve, add the cold-pressed (raw) olive oil. You'll get the benefits of the raw oil and spare yourself the detriments of cooked oils.

⁜ "Sauté" in water instead of oil—you'll just need to stir more.

⁜ On salads, don't give in to the temptation to use bottled dressings. Mix cold-pressed ones such as olive oil, Udo's Choice oil, or flaxseed oil with raw apple cider vinegar. Add spices if you wish.

⁜ Eat foods you are already familiar with, but make them raw. Guacamole and salsa are easy and the recipes are right here in this book (see pages 141 and 143). When you shop for cheeses, look (and ask) for the raw-milk varieties from licensed cheese vendors. If you eat whole-grain breads, you'll love sprouted breads. Get used to finding them in the frozen food section and keeping them in your freezer at home until you're ready to make a sandwich.

⁜ Stay away from highly processed foods like canned gravies and soups and begin reading lists of ingredients on packaged foods. You'll be amazed what sorts of strange additives with unpronounceable names are in what we eat every day. (I get sick just reading them!)

## i already eat a healthy diet. why should i eat raw?

There is what people think is "healthy" and then there is healthy. Within the realm of cooked foods, there are some things that are in my opinion truly deadly. I mean "call 911" deadly. They are the edible version of running out blindly into traffic in the dark of night begging to be mowed down. Guess what? If you invite imminent disaster, you're likely to meet it. High-cholesterol, high-fat, low-fiber diets fall into this category. There are other cooked foods that are usually considered healthy, but in this instance "healthy" is a relative term.

You may be one of those people who is eating what is considered a balanced, low-fat, low-cholesterol diet of cooked food. There is no question that what you're doing is better than stuffing yourself with what's usually referred to as "junk food." But that's still not a *truly* healthy diet. Yes, you're eating a diet of food that is less likely to bring on a heart attack or stroke or liver failure. But that is still merely a lesser of evils. What I'm encouraging is something entirely different. To understand the distinction between cooked food that will keep you alive and raw food that will make you thrive—and it's an essential distinction—read chapter 3. I bet you it will be an eye-opener (and a life saver too).

## when will i start to feel better and look better from eating raw?

You may feel good and look good now—or maybe not—but since what you do to your body is cumulative it is sure to catch up with you over time. What you eat can and almost certainly will have an effect in the future. I believe it's better to tip the odds in your favor than play Russian roulette when it comes to things like your health. Start now by adding raw foods to your diet.

When I started eating raw, I began to feel better almost immediately. My chronic sinus problems were the first to stop bothering me, so the Afrin went. Then I noticed no more stomach problems; indigestion was gone so no more Tums, PeptoBismol, or Mylanta. Then I realized I had not gotten sick that winter—not a cold or a sniffle. So good-bye, NyQuil.

Eating raw changes your body chemistry. Depending on your overall health

when you start you may feel and notice a change right away or it may take a month or more to really notice the difference. In any case, you'll be pleased with the changes in how you feel, how you look, and your outlook on life itself.

## don't you ever get tired of salads? don't you ever get hungry for warm food?

Grrrrrrr! This is perhaps the biggest misconception that people have about eating raw. I'll say it again: I don't eat just cold salads. In fact, I don't even eat mostly salads.

People think that eating raw is all about plates of boring lettuce and celery and carrots. It's not. I would die if I had to eat that way! I eat a wide variety of foods and some of them, though not cooked to the point where the enzymes and proteins are destroyed, are nice and warm. Even if my food is not piping hot, I do drink hot teas or eat soup when I feel the need for heat.

By the way, when you use warming spices like cumin and cayenne, and raw oils, you're sure to feel nice and warm inside even when you're eating raw food.

## eating this way has to be boring. how will i ever get enough to eat?

Since I began eating raw food, I have never been bored with what I eat. Let me tell you why.

Imagine eating a mushroom quiche, spaghetti al pesto, tuna seviche or tartare, portobello stroganoff, apple tarte, lemon custard, fruit parfait topped with whipped cream. Now imagine yourself eating them as often as you need to, without worrying about your weight, and without guilt. That's what I do—I just eat them raw.

No, I don't just eat the uncooked ingredients for these dishes. They are combined into recipes that are beautiful and delicious. Now tell me, does it sound like I'm eating boring food and not getting enough to eat? (The recipes for these and many other raw dishes can be found in chapter 10.)

### if i eat raw to lose weight and then stop eating raw after losing the pounds, will i regain the weight?

You're talking like someone who is going on a diet. If you're like nearly two-thirds of American adults, you're overweight and you have good reason to want to lose weight. So I commend you on wanting to make a change. You should know, however, that yo-yo dieting is a losing battle. The only proven way to overcome obesity and to effectively lose weight and keep it off over the long haul is by making lifestyle changes.

While losing weight is a good motivator for eating raw, I want to encourage you to take a different view. Think of eating raw as having the *secondary* benefit of helping you to lose weight—it is certainly as effective as the best weight-loss plan. Its first benefit, however, is even more important, even if you are over-weight. And that is this: health. You will no longer be putting garbage in your body that tears you down and makes you sick or more prone to being sick. Of course, part of what it does is to make you overweight and being overweight is not healthy. So if you make a lifestyle change that can make you healthier and can cause you to drop the pounds, why would you be asking about changing back to an unhealthy lifestyle?

Though I haven't seen any studies on it, my suspicion is that if you went back to a cooked-food way of life after a period of eating raw I would think you would gain back the weight you've lost. But that still leaves me wondering: if you have every possible satisfying food option open to you as a raw foodist, why would you turn back?

### you're trim and you look so healthy. isn't that mostly just good genes?

There's no question that tall people have an advantage in this world and I'm blessed with "tall genes." But my appearance is directly tied to my eating raw, not to my height. We Alts are not naturally thin. I starved myself for years when I was eating cooked food to help me be thin enough to succeed as a model and actress.

I am now more aware of my body than ever and I feel I can eat what I want

when I want to. I am slimmer and more toned as a result of eating raw food than I ever was when I dieted constantly and ate cooked food. If I have any "genetic advantages," I feel they're enhanced by my eating raw food. I look and feel and I truly am healthier now than I ever have been. That's not a matter of genes. It's a matter of lifestyle. The lifestyle change that has made me this way is eating raw food.

## but what about my family? how can i possibly eat raw food with them around?

Lead the way. If you're eating raw food, others will see the changes in you and your life. They will notice that you're not "on a diet" but that you have made a life change, one that's having a positive effect on you. Besides, you'll be eating all sorts of incredibly delicious foods. They'll be curious and after they get over thinking you must be doing something strange they'll want to have a taste of this or a piece of that. Before too long they're probably going to want you to make certain raw dishes or meals. From there the ball will be rolling.

When I met my boyfriend he had never heard of someone eating raw. He is a professional hockey player. Most athletes I know eat and eat and eat. He ate every kind of cooked food imaginable at all times of day and night. Before too long after we met, he began to ask me about my eating raw food. I told him how raw food had changed my life, dramatically improved my health, and made me feel and look better. I guess he was convinced because despite his playing well he wanted to try raw food. He watched me eat. He and I went out and ate in restaurants together. And very soon he started eating raw too. As an athlete, being sensitive to his body, he sees and feels the difference. He has lost fat and increased muscle definition. In the middle of the season each January he used to get sick, usually with strep. That hasn't happened since eating raw. That's one of the reasons that four years later he's still eating this way.

Don't talk yourself out of eating raw because you don't think your family or friends will understand. Don't fear "sticking out." If you're concerned about not being able to go out with your friends, read what I have to say in chapter 8.

You can do this!

## doesn't it cost a lot?

Garbage is cheap. Junk food is cheap. So of course you can put cheap, worthless garbage into your body and call it "food." What's the result? To me the additional hidden costs of obesity, heart disease, and all sorts of illnesses, not to mention lost productivity, physical discomfort, and the resulting unhappiness. In the end the cost of eating cooked food far outweighs the price you'll pay when you buy healthy food that you can eat raw.

You know what they say: you get what you pay for. When you look at it this way, then you get more for the dollar when you eat raw food than when you eat cooked junk masquerading as food. And by the way, the raw-food restaurants I go to in New York are actually no more expensive, and in some cases less expensive than most of the cooked-food restaurants in town. I also find that now that I eat raw, it takes less food to satisfy me!

## i'm always hungry when i eat salads. they just don't fill me up.

Okay, once again, eating raw is *not* about eating salads, I promise. Don't think "salads" and being hungry. Think satisfaction and being "full" while not feeling guilty for eating. If you try to eat the way I do, you probably won't feel hungry (and you also won't feel fat). So forget the stereotype. Forget salad. But since we're on the subject, let me share with you something Dr. Brantley told me the first time I said to him that I felt hungry when I ate salad: "That's because you eat iceberg lettuce. There are hundreds of veggies that are great tasting and will fill you up because they are nutrient-dense and feed your body." It's true. Iceberg lettuce is really just water in the shape of a leaf. There's not much more to it. Go for the other lettuces, the darker the better. Mix them up with other vegetables and you'll find a salad can be not only more filling but also more tasty and nutritious.

## it may be easy for you to get raw food in new york, but i can't imagine it here in indianapolis.

It's true that my hometown has a higher concentration of raw-food restaurants than any other. In Southern California there are more raw restaurants than in New York but they, like the people, are spread out.

But eating raw is not all about having a place to eat on every corner. It's also not about having to stay home and make dinner every night. Even in Indy you can go out to eat and have a raw dinner (see chapter 8). And when you are eating at home, whether you have a Whole Foods Market on the corner down the block or order on the Internet, you can make and eat countless entirely raw meals that you will love. (Check out chapters 6 and 7 to learn how and chapter 10 for recipes.)

People sometimes think that I'm entirely surrounded by raw foodists who think the way I do or that I'm part of an exclusive club of celebrities who eat raw together all the time. Believe me, neither is the case! But if you eat raw, wherever you are, you'll soon find that others want to try what you're doing, especially as you start to look better. Before you know it you'll have friends who eat raw as well. You'll get together and "un-cook" for one another.

No matter where you live, I believe you can do this. If I could eat raw in Chilliwack, British Columbia, all by myself while working on a movie project, you can eat raw wherever you are, even if you have to ship it in.

## are you saying i need to eat 100 percent raw?

No. I eat almost entirely raw, except for my favorite "cheat," which is the popcorn that I have at hockey games. But eating raw is not an all-or-nothing proposition. Let's face it, there are going to be things you want to eat cooked, even if it may be better for you not to eat them. Well, life shouldn't be so strict that a few guilty pleasures have to be sacrificed.

I remember one day, sitting in a cab in Manhattan, with my friend and writing partner, David Roth. We were at a stop and out the window there was a Vietnamese restaurant. David, who has been to Southeast Asia on several occasions, told me, "Carol, I couldn't eat raw because I couldn't give up Vietnamese and Thai food." I said to him, "Let that be your 'cheat,' your guilty pleasure." He smiled. He had been afraid to get started eating raw because he wasn't ready to go cold turkey. I'll bet he has had pad thai or spring rolls with nuoc mam since that day but he's also eating raw.

Speaking of turkey, if you're an American chances are you celebrate Thanksgiving with the traditional bird in the center of the table and, just like the rest of

the family, a handsome portion on your plate. I like Thanksgiving and so it's my one-time-a-year celebration where I don't concern myself with what I eat. Of course it would be healthier if I skipped the festivities. That's just not practical. And I've tried bringing my own food to the Alt family get-together. It was a disaster. But I don't let Thanksgiving keep me from eating right the rest of the year. I do think taking a few enzyme supplements is a good idea, though—see the Resources for more information.

Don't give up on eating raw because you know you'll be tempted to indulge at holiday times. Just limit what you eat that's not raw and how often you eat it. Give yourself that once-a-week cheat and take enzymes to help you digest. Don't turn the period from Thanksgiving to New Year's into six weeks of recklessly throwing care to the wind. Make some decisions about what you will allow, but remember that there is such a thing as delicious raw pumpkin pie! (Want to make some? Look for the recipe on page 156.) Do the best you can.

Eating raw is not an all-or-nothing proposition. As Dr. Brantley taught me from the start, if you're eating around 70 percent of your food uncooked you'll see a significant change in your health, beauty, mood, and overall well-being. And as you eat more, you'll notice more and more of the positive changes you want. That sort of reinforcement is what I needed to make a permanent, healthy lifestyle change. As best you can, eat it raw. And if you do it, others will follow.

## isn't eating raw food just another fad?

You mean like so many diets? Hardly. I've said it before, but it's worth saying again. Eating raw isn't a diet. It's a way of life, a lifestyle. It's not a weight-loss plan, even though if you have some extra pounds to lose chances are you'll drop them quite easily. People are surprised to learn that what was probably the first all-raw restaurant in America dates back to 1917 when a husband and wife, Vera and John Richter, opened the first of three raw cafeterias called the Eutropheon in Los Angeles. These restaurants lasted for twenty-five years until World War II. And *Eating in the Raw* is hardly the first book on the subject of raw foodism. I encourage you to read other books before making a decision.

Vera Richter published one of America's first uncook books, *Cookless Book,* in 1925. At the same time and living just ten miles away in nearby Van Nuys, Dr. St. Louis A. Estes proclaimed himself the father and founder of the international back-to-nature raw-foods movement. His 1927 book *Raw Food and Health* promotes the merits of raw foods—including dairy products. Nine years later in 1936, John Richter published *Nature the Healer* about the benefits of eating raw, based on a series of his lectures. That's too long ago for this to be a fad.

In my forties, I'm old enough to remember a time when "going jogging" was still considered by some to be a fad, even though there were always people who went running. Well, today tens of millions of people run for fitness, health, and fun. We take running for granted as something that is good for you. And marathon running is booming! Some so-called health fads are not only here to stay, they're becoming mainstream because they deserve to. To me, eating raw is one of them.

### so if eating raw isn't a fad, why have i only recently heard about it?

If the idea of eating raw is new to you you can probably thank the news media for bringing it to your attention. Recently there has been considerable attention brought to raw foodism, attention that was either impossible or unlikely in the past because people just didn't have access to information. Those who were raw foodists were spread out far and wide without real ways to support one another and share their knowledge and experience. But now, with hundreds of channels of TV and radio and especially the Internet, it seems everyone everywhere is connected. Where before you might have to be somewhere like LA to meet raw foodists and to learn about raw food—as I was when I met Dr. Timothy Brantley—now you can find others across town or across the ocean. With the Internet and Web sites like David Wolfe's (a prominent raw-food expert), for example, anyone can learn about how to safely eat raw. You can buy almost any raw food you want online. It's also possible to link up with other people who are eating raw and preparing raw food. There are even Web sites that feature personal ads for raw foodists looking to meet other raw foodists. Like the world

itself, the raw-food world has become a smaller place. It's becoming a global community, and it's growing very quickly. Check out my Web site (www.carol-alt.com) and it will lead you into a whole new raw-food world.

## if it's so good for you and it's not a fad, why do so few people "eat it raw"?

We're creatures of habit and we "follow the leader." In this case, following the leader is doing what the vast majority of humanity does—cook food before eating it. We're at a critical juncture in the history of human eating and, along with it, the way we prepare our foods. You see, we're actually doing something very out of date, very old-fashioned—and I don't mean that in a quaint, nostalgic way—when we eat cooked food. Cooking is a means of preparing foods we use so that we can mix, tenderize, blend, and *keep foods from spoiling before eating them.* But with the development of refrigeration (which, barely a century old, is new in terms of human history) and vacuum sealing (which is even newer), we no longer need to worry so much about spoiling. Still, we do what we have done for ages, what our parents did and what they taught us.

It's going to take some time to undo deep-rooted human habits. But remember that some of us—the Eskimos, for example, and some peoples in the tropics—don't traditionally eat cooked food much, if at all. Humans are the only species that habitually eats cooked food. And I believe it's only a matter of time until our behavior catches up with the possibilities that advances in technology offer us on one hand and with the rest of the animal kingdom's good sense on the other. There has been a boom in interest in health and fitness in recent years. And as more people who are interested in their health begin to learn more about raw food they may start eating raw. It's catching on everywhere now. So why do so few people eat raw? The answer is that I believe more and more *are* doing it all the time! Ask me this question again ten years from now.

## but why aren't there any societies that simply eat raw?

There's a lot we don't know about human origins and even about the customs and behaviors of societies in the days before people started writing things

down. Anthropologists and archaeologists don't know for certain how humans started eating cooked food or when. We don't know exactly where cooking started or how it spread. What we do know, however, includes certain interesting facts. Not everyone eats the same things and cooks the same foods. And not everyone everywhere eats the same amount of cooked food. Traditionally, some peoples eat much more raw food and others eat much less. But until recently, it seemed that the question of whether cooking might not be good for food wasn't often asked. Of course, only recently have we had the scientific means and the interest to investigate and compare what food does in our bodies when it is cooked and when it is raw.

If you have always done something a certain way and you have no reason to question it, you may just keep on doing what you are doing. That's pretty much what we have done with cooking. We just didn't question it. Now that the question is being raised and investigated—and so many people are professing the benefits of raw food—we may become the first generation to make a break with the cooked-food past. With concerns about disease at the forefront of our society today, we may be the first *historical* (but not *pre*historical) society to choose to eat raw.

# 10
## your un- cook book

**recipes for an exciting, satisying, long, and healthy life in the raw**

If you've always been known as a good cook, there's no reason you should give up your reputation in the kitchen just because you're setting aside the pots and pans and turning off the burner. The dishes that follow will not only help you and yours eat life to the fullest, but your friends and family will keep coming back for more—keeping your reputation intact. ✳ Since I started eating raw I've learned a few recipes from friends and family that have become staples in my diet. Along the way I've even created some myself. Some may even

already be familiar to you although you don't necessarily think of them as raw. So whether you're looking for a drink, a snack, a meal, or a dessert, here are some easy-to-prepare menu basics that everyone you know will love. If eating raw is new to you, you can start here, right now.

I've also included some exquisite creations from the kitchens of some outstanding chefs, including a few of the most gifted strictly raw-food chefs out there. They are experts at the craft of not cooking. That's why I look forward to eating whatever they put in front of me every time I sit down in their restaurants. If you love cooking and cherish a gourmet recipe, you'll love these.

## some un-cooking tips

In many ways preparing raw foods is easier than cooking. There are no pots or pans to scrub. There is no preheating the oven and no baked-on mess to soak from the casserole dish. But there are trade-offs. Seeds, nuts, and beans need to be germinated or sprouted to release the nutrients and enzymes and make them digestible. If you eat nuts the way most people do—dry-roasted or honey-roasted, right out of the can—chances are you just chew them up and swallow. They may be tasty that way, but they're not very good for you. Your body needs to be able to fully digest them, something that doesn't happen without soaking them first. And if you're cooking beans rather than sprouting them, you're really missing out on the nutrients that are packed inside. They may taste good, but in my opinion they're not really good for you. Even though they are a protein while raw, they transform into a carbohydrate when cooked.

That means that in your food-preparation plan you have to allow time for soaking and sprouting. I often soak overnight. Start the almonds or chickpeas in the morning, pour off the water at bedtime and when you get up the next day you're ready to make both the morning granola and hummus for lunch or dinner. At the end of the book there's a chart on how long you should soak nuts and beans. The chart will also explain how to sprout alfalfa or other seeds for the freshest possible organic versions of the sprouts you see in the produce department. Just turn to page 165.

On the other hand, a lot of raw dishes can be made quickly and are supposed to be consumed right on the spot after they are made. That's especially true of juices, since the cellular walls of the fruits and vegetables are broken

down to release the nutrients. When the nutrients are exposed to air, they begin to oxidize and deteriorate, so you need to drink them right away.

You need to be careful with animal products if you plan to eat them raw. Always know your sources and specify that you will be eating the meat or fish raw.

If you're wondering about what equipment you'll need for your raw kitchen, it's really quite simple—you'll find that information in chapter 7. And if you're wondering where to get certain ingredients for these recipes, those details are found in chapter 6.

One last reminder: when you go shopping look for the key words *raw* and *organic.* Whenever possible, seek out organic versions of every ingredient in these recipes. Finding raw, organic pantry staples like soy sauce is not an easy task in the average grocery store, and just because you buy some soy sauce in a health-food store does not mean it is both organic and raw. Look for it. You should be able to find it. If you don't, ask if they carry it. If they don't, ask if they'll order it for you. You can also seek out sources on the Internet. Read labels. Ask questions. Why wait to be tired, old, or ill to start eating raw? Have fun. Experiment. *Buon appetito!*

# drinks

## yashin's passion fruit drink

**SERVES 3**

*One night I was experimenting with making a raw drink. My boyfriend walked into the kitchen and sneaked a sip of the base of this drink. He asked if he could add a pinch of this and a bit of that and whatever, and before I knew it he had the frozen berries in hand and had taken over the blender. The result is a fruit drink named after him.*

1 lemon, peeled and seeded

1 pear, cored

10 frozen fresh strawberries

2 bananas

¼ cup apple juice (fresh or unpasteurized)

10 distilled ice cubes

Drop the fruit into the blender, and pour in the juice. Add the ice cubes and blend until smooth.

## almond nut milk

**SERVES 3–5**

*Nut milk is a delicious and nutrient-filled substitute for regular milk. It lasts for a few days in the refrigerator, and stays at its best if vacuum-sealed.*

1 cup germinated almonds (see page 165), or germinated nut of your choice

3–5 cups distilled water

1 tablespoon raw honey

Blend germinated almonds and water until almonds are practically pulverized. Strain through cheesecloth and discard the solids. Blend the liquid with honey.

# too easy (cheater's) almond nut milk

**SERVES 1**

Blend all of the ingredients together in a blender. Adjust the amount of water to achieve the desired thickness.

**2 tablespoons raw almond butter**

**1 teaspoon raw honey**

**1 cup distilled water**

# fresh peach lemonade

**MAKES 1 PITCHER**

*Perfect for a summer party.*

Blend all of the ingredients together in a blender until smooth. Add a few distilled ice cubes if you wish and blend again.

**3 lemons, peeled and seeded**

**1/2 cup raw honey, or to taste**

**1 or 2 peaches, pitted**

**4 cups distilled water**

## simple coconut smoothie

[DAN HOYT AND TOLENTINCHAN, QUINTESSENCE RESTAURANTS,
NEW YORK CITY]

**SERVES 1**

*Some people like to add raw honey. For*
*me, that's just too sweet!*

**1 Thai coconut**

To extract the coconut milk and meat, turn the coconut on its side, and, using a large, sharp knife, trim off the husk of one side to reveal the hard inner shell. Find the three "veins" that run from the center of the coconut. Place the tip of the knife about an inch from the tip of the coconut, between two of the veins. Now tap the knife so that the tip breaks through the shell and goes in about an inch. Next, lower the knife handle so that the blade is parallel to the countertop, making sure that the blade remains at least an inch inside the coconut. Rotate the handle to the left as if you are revving the handles of a motorcycle. Then, rotate the handle to the right. Eventually, by alternating directions, the knife will pry up a piece of the shell. Remove the shell and pour the coconut milk into a bowl. Scoop out the coconut meat with a spoon. An easier way is to get a cleaver (be careful, they're sharp) and just slowly chip away at the one end of the coconut. Pour off the juice and continue chipping until a spoon-size hole is made. Spoon out meat as usual.

Mix the milk and coconut meat in a blender until smooth.

# a breakfast **green drink**

**SERVES 1**

*Green drinks are made with green powder, a nutritionally dense supplement made from various vegetables and other healthy natural ingredients. Some people just stir some "green powder" into unpasteurized apple juice. Here is an easy recipe that's a bit more special. If you are near a Russian or Indian market and can get unpasteurized kefir yogurt, it makes a great addition. Here's to your health.*

**1 banana, peeled**

**1 cup frozen fresh berries**

**2 tablespoons green powder
    (I prefer Quantum Nutrition
    Labs brand)**

**Raw honey, to taste**

Blend the banana, berries, and green powder in a blender until smooth. Stir in raw honey to taste, and enjoy.

# breakfast cereals

## a good start cereal

### SERVES 1

*Start this cereal the night before you want to eat it.*

Grind cereal in a coffee grinder. Transfer to a medium bowl, add enough water to just cover the cereal and let sit overnight. The next morning, add nut milk. Drizzle with raw honey to taste.

**Herb shop organic raw Fourteen-Grain Cereal, as much as you'd like (warning: a little goes a long way)**

**Almond Nut Milk (page 122), to taste**

**Raw honey, to taste**

## oats and fruit cereal

### SERVES 1

*There's no simpler, healthier, raw cereal out there. And it's tasty too!*

Combine all of the ingredients, and enjoy!

**1/2 cup rolled organic oats**

**Almond Nut Milk (page 122), to taste**

**Fresh fruit of your choice**

# david wolfe's basic breakfast granola

**SERVES 4**

Place the softened almonds, raisins, lemon juice, cinnamon, and nutmeg into a blender, and chop until crumbly. Add honey and a drizzle of distilled water. Top it off with Juliano's Whipped Cream or Kelly's Macadamia Whipped Cream, if you like.

**2 cups raw almonds, soaked for 8 hours and drained**

**½ cup raisins**

**2 teaspoons lemon juice**

**1 teaspoon ground cinnamon**

**½ teaspoon ground nutmeg**

**Raw honey, to taste**

**1 tablespoon distilled water (optional)**

**Juliano's Whipped Cream (page 157) or Kelly's Macadamia Whipped Cream (page 155) (optional)**

# peter clement's cholesterol-busting morning granola

**SERVES 4**

Place the softened almonds, raisins, walnuts, lemon juice, and cinnamon into a blender, and chop till crumbly. Mix in the oats. Add nut milk or water to moisten. Drizzle with honey, if you like it sweet, and serve with fruit, if you wish.

**2 cups raw almonds, soaked for 8 hours and drained**

**½ cup raisins**

**½ handful raw, germinated walnut pieces (page 165)**

**Juice of 1 lemon**

**1 teaspoon ground cinnamon**

**¼–½ cup organic rolled oats**

**¼–½ cup Almond Nut Milk (page 122) or distilled water**

**Raw honey, to taste**

**Fresh fruit (optional)**

# soups

## marvelous **miso broth**

**SERVES 1**

*Unpasteurized, organic miso is a delicious, versatile fermented soybean paste. It comes in different "flavors," from a mellow yellow variety to deeper, more pungent red and brown types. You should find the miso in the refrigerated foods section of large supermarkets, health-food stores, and Asian markets year-round.*

**1 teaspoon unpasteurized miso paste (your favorite variety)**

**2 teaspoons Bragg Liquid Aminos, or to taste**

**1 cup distilled water**

**Seaweed, sliced carrots, and/or mushrooms, to taste**

Mix the miso with Bragg Liquid Aminos. Bring the water to a boil, and pour it over the miso and Bragg mixture. Add more Bragg Liquid Aminos if you'd like the broth to be saltier. Drop in the seaweed, carrots, and/or mushrooms.

# gazpacho

**SERVES 4**

Place the pepper, tomatoes, onion, garlic, water, vinegar, lemon juice, cucumber, and cilantro in a blender, and puree. Strain to remove any vegetable pieces that are not fully liquefied. Chill overnight, if time permits. Before serving, sprinkle the chopped scallion over the top of the gazpacho.

**1 green bell pepper, seeded, cored, and diced**

**4 tomatoes, diced**

**1 medium white onion, diced**

**3 garlic cloves, peeled and minced**

**3 cups distilled water**

**Raw apple cider vinegar, to taste**

**Freshly squeezed lemon juice, to taste**

**1 cucumber, peeled and chopped (optional)**

**4 tablespoons freshly chopped cilantro (optional)**

**1 scallion (green part), finely chopped, for garnish**

# seventh heaven soup

[DAVID JUBB, JUBB'S LONGEVITY, NEW YORK CITY]

**SERVES 4**

*I met David Jubb at Quintessence Restaurant one day when* Inside Edition *was filming a story on eating raw that featured raw-food personality David Wolfe, actress/chef Leslie Bega, and myself. In strolled this amazing, different-looking man, so full of fun and life and light— David Jubb. Everyone in Quintessence was shocked I didn't know him. "You don't know David Jubb?" "You've never been to Jubb's Longevity?" "You've got to taste his food." So I invited Jubb to be interviewed for* Inside Edition *and then went over to taste his food and was hooked immediately. Here is one of Jubb's truly extraordinary raw recipes.*

½ cup sesame seeds

1 cucumber, unpeeled

1 red bell pepper, seeded and cored

2 celery stalks

1 medium tomato

¼ cup chopped red onion

1 apple, cored

1-inch knob fresh gingerroot, peeled

3 garlic cloves, peeled

1–2 bushy sprigs fresh cilantro

¼ cup freshly squeezed lemon juice

2½ cups distilled water

2 heaping tablespoons unpasteurized miso

¼ cup Bragg Liquid Aminos

**TOPPING**

¼ cup cold-pressed flaxseed or olive oil

¼ teaspoon ground cayenne pepper (optional)

½ teaspoon minced garlic

Spirulina flakes, for garnish

Grind the sesame seeds to a moist meal in your spice grinder; it takes only a few seconds. Cut the vegetables and apple into chunks, and place in a blender. Add the gingerroot and garlic, and blend with the cilantro, lemon juice, water, miso, and Bragg Liquid Aminos to make the gazpacho. Depending on how much gusto your blender has, you may have to shred harder vegetables and blend in two batches, especially if the blender container is on the small side.

To make the topping, blend all of the topping ingredients together in a small bowl. Ladle the gazpacho into bowls, and drizzle with the flavored-oil topping. Garnish the soup with some spirulina flakes.

## spirulina

Although you may never have heard of it, spirulina has nourished people in Africa and America throughout the ages. Only recently have scientists discovered the health benefits that indigenous peoples have depended on for centuries. This microalgae is 60% all-vegetable protein. It is rich in beta-carotene, iron, vitamin $B_{12}$, and an array of other vitamins, minerals, and phytonutrients as well as the rare essential fatty acid, GLA (gamma-linolenic acid). You can find spirulina flakes in any health-food store.

# salads and dressings

## tatiana's **game time greens**

**SERVES 2**

*This salad is especially healthful if you use Udo's Choice oil, a special blend of cold-pressed oils that provide the perfect balance of essential fatty acids that every body needs. It's available in the refrigerated section of many health-food stores—if you can't find it, ask for it!*

Combine mesclun greens and other vegetables in a large bowl. Add the olives and cheese. Drizzle with both oils, toss, and season with salt and pepper. Toss in the avocado chunks and sprinkle with cayenne pepper.

- 1 4.5-ounce bag organic mesclun salad
- 1 cucumber, peeled and thinly sliced
- 1 tomato, diced
- 1 green, yellow, or red bell pepper, seeded, cored, and thinly sliced
- 5 raw olives (preferably Nature's First Law), pitted and halved
- 1 ounce raw-milk goat cheese, sliced or crumbled
- $2/3$ cup cold-pressed olive oil
- $1/3$ cup Udo's Choice oil
- Sea salt, to taste
- Freshly ground black pepper, to taste
- 1 avocado, pitted and diced (optional)
- Ground cayenne pepper, to taste

# marybeth's raw broccoli salad

**SERVES 8**

*I went to a New York Islanders summer party where one of the executives' wives served this amazing salad. When I asked her for the ingredients I knew I could make it raw. So she sent me the recipe and I looked for raw substitutions—mostly because the ramen soup seasoning she used in the dressing listed salt and MSG as its first two ingredients! So here's Mary-beth's party salad, with a raw variation on the dressing that I think is even tastier and infinitely better for you.*

1½ pounds broccoli

1 bunch scallions (green parts only), chopped

1 cup raw slivered germinated almonds (see page 165)

1 cup raw germinated sunflower seeds (see page 165)

**DRESSING**

4 pitted dates

1 tablespoon distilled water

¾ cup raw apple cider vinegar

¼ cup Udo's Choice oil (see page 132)

¼ cup cold-pressed extra-virgin olive oil

Slice the broccoli into thin strips as you would cabbage for cole slaw. Toss the broccoli, scallions, slivered almonds, and sunflower seeds together in a large bowl and set aside.

To make the dressing, put the dates and water in a blender. Blend to create a coarse paste. Add the vinegar and oils, and blend again to emulsify. Pour the dressing over the salad and toss to combine.

# "tuna" salad

[DAN HOYT AND TOLENTIN CHAN, QUINTESSENCE RESTAURANTS, NEW YORK CITY]

**SERVES 6**

*One morning about 2 years ago, the* New York Post *called, asking if I would do a personal favor and, since I was a raw-food eater, take a photo for them at Quintessence, a raw-food restaurant. I was shocked. A raw-food restaurant? I didn't even know they existed. I had to go.*

*That's how I met Dan Hoyt, the owner of Quintessence. He prepared several dishes for us to photograph. So I was lucky—I got to taste test, for free, all of Dan's dishes. Now I'm a regular—and my photo hangs in the entrance! Here is one of my favorite Quintessence dishes.*

Combine the walnuts, dulse, herbs, garlic, lemon juice, oil, and salt in the bowl of a food processor, using the "S" blade. Transfer to a large mixing bowl, and stir in the celery, pepper, and onion.

**"TUNA" SALAD**

**2 cups raw, germinated walnuts (page 165)**

**¼ cup dulse (red seaweed), soaked for 10 minutes, and drained**

**4 tablespoons chopped fresh dill**

**4 tablespoons chopped fresh parsley**

**2 garlic cloves**

**½ cup freshly squeezed lemon juice**

**¼ cup cold-pressed olive oil**

**2 teaspoons sea salt**

**2–3 celery stalks, chopped**

**1 red bell pepper, seeded, cored, and chopped**

**½ medium white onion, chopped**

# lentil salad

**SERVES 4**

*Don't forget—to best unlock the nutrients in those hard and stubborn lentils, germinate them for 8 hours!*

Mix the germinated lentils, onion, optional tomato, and cucumber in a medium bowl. Pour the oils and vinegar over the lentil salad, and toss well. Season with sea salt and a squeeze of lemon. Toss again. Let sit for 2 to 3 hours in the refrigerator to absorb the nice onion flavor.

**1 cup raw germinated lentils (see page 165)**

**1 chopped white onion**

**1 tomato, chopped**

**1 cucumber, chopped**

**2 tablespoons Udo's Choice oil (see page 132)**

**2 tablespoons cold-pressed extra-virgin olive oil**

**⅛ cup raw apple cider vinegar (optional)**

**Sea salt, to taste**

**¼ lemon (optional)**

# martin's favorite cole slaw

**SERVES 4**

*David, my writer, was trying out different recipes on his kids, and since he has five of them, they don't always agree on food. But all of them say this salad is David's finest (and it's named for his youngest son).*

Mix all of the ingredients together in a large bowl, and serve.

1 cup shredded red cabbage

1 cup shredded green cabbage

½ carrot, shredded

¼ cup shredded white onion

1 tablespoon cumin seeds

Juice from 1 lemon

1 teaspoon Celtic sea salt

2 garlic cloves, minced

1 teaspoon ground cumin

⅓ cup cold-pressed extra-virgin olive oil

Drizzle of raw cider vinegar

1 medium tomato, diced (optional)

# caesar salad

**SERVES 4**

*I love caesar salad and even order it at restaurants when I go out—although I take lots of enzymes to counteract the cooked olive oil and un-raw-milk parmesan and I avoid the wheat-filled croutons. When I eat this at home, I don't need enzymes—I just enjoy.*

Rub garlic into the inside of a large wooden salad bowl. Place the lettuce in the bowl. In a medium mixing bowl, combine all the dressing ingredients. Add the dressing to the romaine lettuce in the salad bowl, and toss to combine.

**1 garlic clove, chopped**

**2 heads organic romaine lettuce, chopped into bite-size pieces**

**DRESSING**

**½ cup grated raw milk Parmesan or Pecorino-Romano cheese**

**½ cup cold-pressed extra-virgin olive oil**

**¼ cup raw apple cider vinegar**

**1 fertile, organic egg**

**2 tablespoons Bragg Liquid Aminos**

**Juice of ½ lemon**

# carol's simplest salad dressing

**MAKES 2³/₄ CUPS**

Put all of the ingredients in a plastic container with lid. Shake well. For added pleasure and zing, add mustard powder and a splash more oil to make a mustard vinaigrette. (Sometimes I cheat and add Dijon.)

1 cup Udo's Choice oil (see page 132)

1 cup cold-pressed extra-virgin olive oil

¾ cup raw apple cider vinegar

Sea salt, to taste

Ground cayenne pepper (optional)

Ground mustard, to taste

# jubb's dill dijon dressing

**MAKES 1¼ CUPS**

*Here's a more involved mustard dressing.*

Blend all of the ingredients in a blender.

3–4 tablespoons Dijon mustard

3 tablespoons Shoyu (unpasteurized soy sauce)

¼ cup raw apple cider vinegar

1 tablespoon raw tahini

¼ cup cold-pressed olive oil

½ lemon, juiced

3 bushy sprigs fresh dill or 3 tablespoons dried dill

1 tablespoon honey or raisins

¼ cup distilled water

# sandwiches

## the **hungry man sandwich**

**SERVES 1**

*Most breads that I recommend, like Manna, Ezekiel, and Genesis, are not truly raw. But because they are sprouted, they at least don't have potentially harmful gluten. The only truly raw breads I've found are in raw-food restaurants and specialty shops.*

Sprinkle the bread with oil and season with salt and cayenne. Spread the smashed avocado on top, and season with more sea salt and cayenne pepper. Lay slices of the cheese on the avocado, and add lettuce leaves and tomato slices.

**2 slices Ezekiel or Genesis bread**

**Cold-pressed olive oil, flaxseed oil, and/or Udo's Choice oil (see page 132)**

**Sea salt, to taste**

**Ground cayenne pepper, to taste**

**½ avocado, pitted and smashed**

**Raw sheep's milk cheese (raw goat's milk or raw cow's milk cheese can be substituted)**

**Lettuce leaves (green leaf, red leaf, or Boston)**

**Tomato slices**

# muriel's start 'em young sandwich

**SERVES 1**

Spread the almond butter on the bread. Add banana slices and strawberries, if you like.

**Raw Almond Nut Butter (storebought, or use the recipe below)**

**2 slices Ezekiel or Genesis bread**

**1 ripe banana, sliced**

**Sliced strawberries (optional)**

# almond nut butter

**MAKES ABOUT 1 CUP**

*This is great for sandwiches! Of course, it's even easier to buy raw nut butter at a natural-foods store or at Whole Foods.*

Grind almonds in the food processor until they form a paste. Blend in the water and oil, and stir in the sea salt.

**1 cup raw almonds, soaked for 8 hours and drained**

**5–6 tablespoons distilled water**

**1 tablespoon Udo's Choice oil (see page 132)**

**Pinch of sea salt**

# snacks and hors d'oeuvres

## carol's **everyday guacamole**

**SERVES 3**

Scoop the meat from the avocado skins. Cut the avocados into chunks, place in a large bowl, and mash with a spoon. Gently stir in the onions, tomatoes, and cilantro. Squeeze in the lime juice, and stir in salt to taste.

**3 avocados, pitted**

**1 red onion, diced**

**2 tomatoes, diced**

**2 sprigs fresh cilantro, finely chopped**

**1 lime**

**Sea salt, to taste**

# raw hummus

**SERVES 4**

*This recipe really makes you love your Vitamix. I burned out five blenders until I finally broke down and bought one!*

In a blender, puree the chickpeas with ½ cup oil. Gradually blend in the remaining ½ cup oil. Add water to reach the desired thickness. When creamy, blend in the tahini, then the lemon juice. Keep blending until creamy again. Add garlic and blend again. Season with salt. You can eat the hummus right away, but it's always best a few hours later.

**3 cups raw germinated chickpeas (see page 165)**

**1 cup cold-pressed olive oil or Udo's Choice oil**

**Distilled water as needed**

**½ cup raw tahini with its oil**

**Juice of ½ lemon**

**1 garlic clove, chopped**

**Sea salt, to taste**

# salsa

**MAKES ABOUT 1 1/2 CUPS**

*Great with raw flaxseed crackers (try the ones by Nature's First Law) and Genesis or Ezekiel bread.*

Combine the pepper, tomato, onion, garlic, cilantro, lemon juice, and oil in a medium bowl, and toss to fully blend. Season with salt and jalapeño to taste.

1 green bell pepper, seeded, cored, and diced

1 tomato, diced

1/2 red onion, diced

1 garlic clove, chopped

2 sprigs fresh cilantro, finely chopped

Juice of 1/4 lemon

1/4 cup cold-pressed olive oil or Udo's Choice oil

Sea salt, to taste

Chopped jalapeño pepper, to taste

# nature's first law **olive paste**

**MAKES 3/4–1 CUP**

*Spread on flaxseed crackers or Ezekiel bread for hors d'oeuvres.*

Puree the olives in a blender, adding enough juice from the olive jar to achieve desired thickness.

1 13-ounce jar pitted raw olives (preferably Nature's First Law Italian)

# entrées

## portobello stroganoff

[DAVID JUBB, JUBB'S LONGEVITY, NEW YORK CITY]

**SERVES 6**

Combine the portobellos, onion, zucchini, bell peppers, jalapeño, vinegar, honey, oil, tahini, water, and herbs and spices in a large pot and heat just to 118 degrees F. on an instant-read thermometer, or until just warm to the touch. Make a bed of shredded lettuce on each plate. Pour the warmed, but not cooked, sauce over the shredded romaine lettuce beds. Garnish with asparagus and nasturtiums for color.

**5 portobello mushroom caps, sliced**

**1 yellow onion, sliced**

**3 zucchini, sliced**

**2 red bell peppers, seeded and sliced**

**1 jalapeño, seeded and sliced**

**¼ cup raw apple cider vinegar or lemon juice**

**2 tablespoons raw honey**

**1 cup cold-pressed olive oil**

**4 teaspoons raw tahini**

**5 cups distilled water**

**2 sprigs fresh rosemary, chopped**

**2 teaspoons kelp or dulse powder**

**4 teaspoons curry powder**

**1 teaspoon sea salt**

**2 teaspoons freshly ground black pepper**

**1 head romaine lettuce, shredded**

**½ pound asparagus spears, lightly blanched, for garnish**

**Nasturtium flowers, for garnish**

# sushi samba **tuna seviche**

[SUSHI SAMBA, NEW YORK CITY]

**SERVES 4**

*This dish, by chefs Takanori Wada and Robert Ash, is one of my favorites at Sushi Samba. The key to preparing and eating raw fish yourself is to find a reputable fish market or a gourmet grocery where you can be certain you're getting the freshest catch. Be sure to ask for "sushi-grade" fish. If you don't know where to get sushi-grade fish, call around. If a fish-market manager knows you're going to want something on a certain day, he or she may be able to order it for you and have it fresh. This is one type of raw food that is going to be much easier to find on or near the coasts than in the heartland.*

**¾ pound sushi-grade bigeye tuna, thinly sliced**

**¼ cup red onion, thinly sliced**

**¼ cup celery, thinly sliced**

**¼ cup red and/or yellow bell peppers, thinly sliced**

**½ fresh jalapeño, thinly sliced**

**4 teaspoons scallions (green and white parts), finely chopped**

**Chives, for garnish**

**SEVICHE MARINADE**

**1 cup freshly squeezed orange juice**

**½ cup freshly squeezed lemon juice**

**½ cup freshly squeezed lime juice**

**¼ cup raw soy sauce (*nama shoyu*)**

**¾ cup raw olive oil**

**1 tablespoon minced garlic**

**1 tablespoon peeled minced fresh gingerroot**

**Salt and freshly ground black pepper, to taste**

Chill the prepared fish and vegetables in separate bowls.

To make the seviche marinade, combine all the ingredients, mix well, and refrigerate for at least 1 hour.

To assemble, lay out 4 chilled salad plates, combine seviche marinade with the tuna and vegetables, mix well, and spoon equal amounts of seviche onto salad plates.

I prefer to marinate the fish in the sauce.

**See photograph on back cover.**

# doctor minarik's ceviche royal

**SERVES 6**

*When I was eating at Quintessence, I came across a pamphlet on a naturopath, Dr. Minarek. It explained how he cured Mohammed Ali of his ailments while boxing and rid Jackie O of a chronic neck problem—all by foot reflexology. Minarek had been around! So I thought "Why not? I loved to have my feet massaged." It was a terrific move because now, in addition to the reflexology, Dr. Minarek is always trying new recipes on me. This one is a favorite.*

In a large bowl, combine the tomatoes, onion, herbs and spices, lemon and lime juices, and soy sauce. Gently fold in the cubed salmon, sea bass, scallops, and let marinate in the refrigerator for 3 hours before serving.

½ pint grape tomatoes

1 medium purple onion, chopped

1 bunch fresh cilantro (leaves only)

1 heaping tablespoon vegetable and herb powder mix

1 tablespoon garlic powder

⅛ teaspoon ground cayenne pepper

1 teaspoon evaporated Celtic sea salt

Juice of 2 lemons

Juice of 15 limes

2 tablespoons raw soy sauce (*nama shoyu*)

1 pound sushi-grade salmon, cubed

1 pound sushi-grade Chilean sea bass, cubed

1 pound sushi-grade bay scallops, cubed

# tuna tartare

[LENOX ROOM, NEW YORK CITY]

**SERVES 2**

*When Charlie Palmer, Tony Fortuna, and Edward Bianchini opened the Lenox Room it was all the buzz in New York—and for good reason. Not only are these three of the most accomplished restaurateurs in town, but they also brought chefs Andrew Thompson and Matthew Geraghty under the same roof to create an American cuisine with French accents—and they installed a distinctive raw bar. How could a raw foodist like me resist? A far cry from a health-food restaurant, the Lenox serves something for everyone, including me. Here's my favorite item on their menu, Tuna Tartare.*

Mix the tuna, chives, shallots, gingerroot, cumin, cayenne pepper, soy sauce, oil, and sesame seeds. Place a neat mound of tartare on each plate. Garnish with sesame oil, scallions, and mixed greens.

**1 pound sushi-grade yellowfin tuna, diced**

**3 tablespoons fresh chives, chopped**

**3 tablespoons shallots, chopped**

**2 tablespoons chopped peeled fresh gingerroot**

**2 teaspoons ground cumin**

**1/2 teaspoon ground cayenne pepper**

**2 tablespoons raw soy sauce (*nama shoyu*)**

**3 tablespoons cold-pressed extra-virgin olive oil**

**1 tablespoon black and/or white sesame seeds**

**A drizzle of raw sesame oil (if you can't find it, use the oil off the top of a can of raw tahini), for garnish**

**Chopped scallions, for garnish**

**Mixed greens, for garnish**

# quiche aux champignons (mushroom quiche)

[KELLY SERBONICH, HIPPOCRATES HEALTH INSTITUTE,
WEST PALM BEACH, FLORIDA]

**SERVES 4**

*Founded more than four decades ago by Ann Wigmore as a center to promote wellness through natural means, the Hippocrates Health Institute is an icon in the raw-food world. Today its executive chef is a radiant twenty-something named Kelly Serbonich who started her career in food at age sixteen by flipping burgers and making fries. After earning a degree in culinary arts, she studied nutrition and ended up a raw foodist. Combining her artistry as a chef with her knowledge of nutrition and a commitment to the benefits of eating raw, Serbonich's food draws people to southern Florida from all over the globe. Here is one of her favorite creations, all of which have her characteristic French flair.*

In the bowl of a food processor, combine all of the crust ingredients. Process until a dough is formed and the walnuts are very well chopped. Season with salt and pepper. Very lightly oil a 12-inch pie pan or dish. Press the crust mixture into the plate and dehydrate overnight, or let sit in the sun for 1 to 4 hours.

### CRUST

**3 cups raw, germinated walnuts (page 165)**

**¼ cup flaxseeds, ground**

**1 garlic clove**

**½ teaspoon dried thyme or herbs de Provence**

**½ teaspoon dried tarragon**

**½ tablespoon Bragg Liquid Aminos**

**Salt and freshly ground black pepper, to taste**

### FILLING

**¾ cup chopped scallions (green and white parts)**

**3½ cups chopped cremini mushrooms**

**⅓ cup cold-pressed extra-virgin olive oil**

**2 tablespoons Bragg Liquid Aminos**

**Juice of 1½ lemons**

**Pinch of ground nutmeg**

**1 cup raw, germinated walnuts (page 165) or 1 cup tahini**

**1½ teaspoons psyllium husks powder**

**1 cup distilled water**

To make the filling, marinate the chopped scallions and mushrooms in olive oil and $\frac{1}{2}$ tablespoon Bragg Liquid Aminos in a large bowl for at least 1 hour.

In a blender, combine the lemon juice, nutmeg, walnuts or tahini, psyllium powder, water, and the remaining $1\frac{1}{2}$ tablespoons of Braggs Liquid Aminos. Blend well until smooth and creamy. Fold this mixture into the marinated mushrooms and scallions. Spread evenly over the crust. Chill for at least 1 hour and serve. The quiche will firm up as it sits.

# spaghetti al pesto

[QUINTESSENCE, NEW YORK CITY]

**SERVES 3**

Thinly slice the yellow squash with a sharp knife, or, better yet, use a turning (spiralizing) slicer (see page 85) to create strands of "pasta." Set aside. For the pesto sauce, put all the ingredients in a blender and blend until creamy. Toss the pesto sauce with the sliced or spiralized squash pasta and serve.

**See photograph on back cover.**

**3 pounds yellow summer squash**

**PESTO SAUCE**

**1 cup pine nuts**

**1 cup cold-pressed olive oil**

**½ large bunch fresh basil**

**½ cup chopped fresh parsley**

**3 garlic cloves**

**1 teaspoon evaporated sea salt**

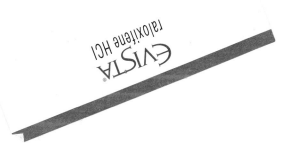

# pasta **alla marinara**

[QUINTESSENCE, NEW YORK CITY]

**SERVES 5**

For the "pasta," thinly slice the yellow squash with a sharp knife, or, better yet, use a turning (spiralizing) slicer (see page 85) to cut squash into curly strands. Set aside. For the marinara sauce, put all the sauce ingredients in a blender and puree until creamy. Pour sauce on spiralized yellow squash pasta and top with olives, tomatoes, bell peppers, and onions.

A "parmesan cheese" may be made by putting an equal proportion of sea salt and raw sesame seeds in a coffee grinder and blending until flaky, like the consistency of ground parmesan.

**5 pounds yellow summer squash**

**MARINARA SAUCE**

**6 large tomatoes**

**½ cup sundried tomatoes**

**2 garlic cloves**

**½ bunch fresh basil**

**¼ cup (loosely packed) fresh oregano**

**2 tablespoons chopped fresh tarragon**

**2 tablespoons chopped fresh rosemary**

**2 tablespoons chopped fresh sage**

**1 tablespoon freshly ground black pepper**

**¼ cup red onion, chopped**

**½ cup cold-pressed olive oil**

**¼ cup lemon juice**

**5 dates, pitted**

**1 tablespoon evaporated sea salt**

**TOPPING**

**¼ cup olives, chopped**

**¼ cup tomatoes, chopped**

**¼ cup red bell peppers, chopped**

**¼ cup red onions, chopped**

# desserts

## fruit parfait

*This one's too easy.*

For each serving, place a layer of whipped cream into a parfait glass, add a layer of granola, then a layer of fruit, followed by another layer of whipped cream, granola, fruit, and a final dollop of whipped cream.

**Kelly's Macadamia Whipped Cream (page 155)**

**Fresh fruit (berries are nice!)**

**Basic Breakfast Granola (page 127)**

## watermelon sorbet

**SERVES 5**

*This one's even easier!*

Scoop out watermelon flesh; then puree it until thoroughly liquefied. Add water until the watermelon sorbet has the desired consistency. Transfer to ice-cube trays and freeze. Once frozen, reblend the frozen watermelon cubes in the blender, adding a little lemon juice to taste. You're done!

**Distilled water, to taste**

**Organic watermelon**

**Freshly squeezed lemon juice, to taste**

# manna from heaven

*Manna bread is also called Essene bread (after the desert sect that produced the Dead Sea Scrolls and John the Baptist is believed to have belonged to). It is a highly nutritious, sprouted bread that is baked at very low temperatures; even though it is not raw, much of its nutritional value remains intact. You'll find this bread in the frozen-food section of better supermarkets and, of course, in health food stores. There are several brands and, at last count, six different kinds: rye, sunflower seed, multigrain, cinnamon raison, nut and date, and carrot. The first three are best with cheeses and for dinner; the last three make a delicious, simple dessert . . . as in this recipe.*

**Manna bread slices**

**Raw honey, to taste**

**Raw germinated almonds (see page 165), to taste**

Lay out the slices of manna bread. Drizzle raw honey on the bread. Grind some almonds and sprinkle on top. Eat open-faced. Heavenly!

# kelly's unbaked apples

[KELLY SERBONICH, HIPPOCRATES HEALTH INSTITUTE,
WEST PALM BEACH, FLORIDA]

**SERVES 4**

*By the way, this stuffing is also excellent in halved pears, again topped with Kelly's Macadamia Whipped Cream.*

Place the apples in the dehydrator for approximately 24 hours, or until desired doneness is achieved.

In the bowl of a food processor, combine the walnuts, raisins, vanilla extract, cinnamon, cloves, and dates. Process to a crumble. Stuff the mixture in the apples and dehydrate again until warm and crunchy. I'll leave it up to you to be the judge. Top with Kelly's Macadamia Whipped Cream.

**4 apples, halved with the middle hollowed out**

**1 cup raw germinated walnuts (see page 165)**

**½ cup raisins, soaked and drained**

**1 tablespoon alcohol-free vanilla extract**

**1½ teaspoon ground cinnamon**

**Pinch of ground cloves**

**4 dates, pitted and chopped**

**Kelly's Macadamia Whipped Cream (recipe follows) to serve**

# kelly's macadamia whipped cream

**MAKES 2 CUPS**

In a strong blender, combine all ingredients. Blend until smooth and creamy. Use as a topping for pies, beverages, puddings, and so on.

**1 cup macadamia nuts, soaked for 8–10 hours and dehydrated in a dehydrator overnight**

**½ cup Thai coconut water (see page 124)**

**5 dates, pitted and soaked**

**1 tablespoon organic cold-pressed coconut butter**

# kelly's lemon custard

**SERVES 3**

In a strong blender, combine all ingredients and blend until very smooth. Check for flavor, and add more dates or lemon juice accordingly. Pour into serving/molding cups and chill. Garnish with strawberries or kiwi and serve.

**2 cups Thai coconut meat (see page 124)**

**5 tablespoons freshly squeezed lemon juice**

**1 cup Thai coconut water**

**8 dates, pitted and soaked**

**½ teaspoon psyllium husks powder**

**1 tablespoon alcohol-free vanilla extract**

**3 strawberries or 1 sliced kiwi, for garnish**

## the *eating in the raw*
# thanksgiving pumpkin pie
[QUINTESSENCE, NEW YORK CITY]

**SERVES 8**

For the crust, put the crust ingredients in a blender and grind until coarse. Scoop out and press into an oiled 12-inch pie pan.

For the filling, combine the filling ingredients in a blender. The consistency of the filling at room temperature should be like that of a batter. If it's too thin, add a few more almonds and puree again. Pour the filling into the crust and refrigerate for 2 hours or preferably overnight. The pie will firm up.

To serve, slice the chilled pie into wedges and top with Kelly's Macadamia Whipped Cream or Juliano's Whipped Cream.

**See photograph on back cover.**

**CRUST**

**2 cups raw germinated almonds (see page 165)**

**1/2 cup dried, shredded raw coconut (optional)**

**Juice of 1 lemon**

**1 teaspoon ground cinnamon**

**1/2 teaspoon ground nutmeg**

**FILLING**

**2 cups cubed ripe raw pumpkin (without seeds)**

**1 1/4 cup raw germinated almonds (see page 165)**

**2 tablespoons freshly squeezed orange juice**

**2 organic, fertile egg yolks (optional)**

**2 tablespoons raw honey**

**1/2 teaspoon ground ginger**

**1 teaspoon ground cinnamon**

**1/4 teaspoon ground nutmeg**

**1/2 teaspoon alcohol-free vanilla extract**

**TOPPING**

**Kelly's Macadamia Whipped Cream (page 155), or Juliano's Whipped Cream (page 157)**

# juliano's **whipped cream**

[JULIANO, *RAW THE UNCOOK BOOK,* SANTA MONICA, CALIFORNIA]

**MAKES ABOUT 2 CUPS**

*Juliano is the epitome of a colorful char-acter and is probably the most well-known raw chef around. His beautifully illus-trated book,* Raw: The Uncook Book, *set a new standard for raw-food recipe books and convinced more than a few skeptics that raw food could be as delicious and look as beautiful as anything they had ever had cooked. Here's the simplest of all Juliano recipes, and one that proves that less can be more than you might ever anticipate. Here's Juliano's easy-to-make, very versatile, and utterly scrumptious whipped cream.*

**1 1/2 cups raw germinated walnuts, cashews, or nuts of your choice (see page 165)**

**1/3 cup freshly squeezed orange juice**

**2 tablespoons dates, chopped**

**A few drops of almond extract (optional)**

In a blender, combine the nuts, orange juice, dates, and, if you wish, a few drops of almond extract. Blend, and using a rubber scraper, scrape the sides to help the cream blend. Stop and check for sweetness and consistency; add more chopped dates if the cream needs sweetness; add more water if the cream is still too stiff. Continue blending until fluffy and smooth. Use immediately.

# tarte aux pommes (apple tart)

[KELLY SERBONICH, HIPPOCRATES HEALTH INSTITUTE, WEST PALM BEACH, FLORIDA]

**SERVES 8**

*Delicious as is, this tart can also be served with Crème Anglaise (page 159).*

To make the crust, use the S blade in a food processor to finely grind the almonds and hazelnuts to a crumbly powder. Add the cinnamon, apricots, and Bragg Liquid Aminos, if using. Process until the mixture begins to ride up the sides of the food processor. Use a little coconut oil to lubricate a 12-inch tart pan or pie plate so that the crust will not stick after dehydrating. Press the crust to an even thickness inside the tart pan or pie plate.

To make the filling, in the bowl of a food processor, combine all the filling ingredients. Process well, until an applesauce-like mixture is achieved. Spread this mixture evenly over the crust.

**CRUST**

- 1 cup germinated almonds (see page 165)
- 1 cup hazelnuts, soaked for 8–10 hours and dehydrated in a dehydrator overnight
- ½ teaspoon ground cinnamon
- 8 dried apricots, soaked for 15 minutes, liquid reserved
- ½ teaspoon Bragg Liquid Aminos (optional)
- Raw coconut oil, for pan

**FILLING**

- 1¾ cups roughly chopped apples
- 20 dried apricots, soaked in water for 15 minutes
- 1 tablespoon alcohol-free vanilla extract
- 4 dates, pitted and soaked for 15 minutes
- 1 tablespoon organic cold-pressed coconut butter (optional)
- ¼ cup apricot soaking liquid
- 1 teaspoon psyllium husks powder
- ½ teaspoon ground cinnamon

To make the topping, toss the apples with the lemon juice and vanilla extract in a mixing bowl. Decoratively lay the sliced apples atop the applesauce mixture. Dehydrate overnight for a "baked" look.

To make the glaze, blend the apricot soaking liquid and psyllium to create a smooth mixture. Brush the glaze on the tart before serving.

**TOPPING**

**1¹/₂ cups apples, peeled, cored, and thinly sliced**

**Juice from ¹/₂ lemon**

**¹/₂ tablespoon alcohol-free vanilla extract**

**GLAZE**

**¹/₄ cup reserved apricot soaking liquid**

**¹/₂ teaspoon psyllium husks powder**

# kelly's crème anglaise

**MAKES 3 CUPS**

*This also makes a good ice-cream mixture. Just freeze in an ice cream machine and enjoy!*

In a strong blender, combine all the ingredients. Blend very well until very smooth. Use additional date soaking liquid or coconut water to adjust the consistency if necessary.

**4 dates, soaked in water for 15 minutes (liquid reserved)**

**1 cup Thai coconut meat (see page 124)**

**1¹/₂ tablespoons alcohol-free vanilla extract**

**A few drops of your favorite flavored extract (optional)**

**²/₃ cup reserved date soaking liquid, or Thai coconut water (page 124)**

# banana tiramisù

[A. J. HILL AND SUNSHINE PHELPS, FOOD WITHOUT FIRE,
MIAMI BEACH, FLORIDA]

**SERVES 6**

*Having spent so much time in Italy over the years, I really enjoy a first-rate tiramisu for dessert. Imagine how pleased I was when I decided to get away to southern Florida in the dead of winter and discovered a wonderful little place to eat raw: Food Without Fire—and their amazing Banana Tiramisù. Rated 10+ by two Italians!*

**"LADYFINGER" CRUST**

**2 cups raw pecans**

**¹⁄₂ cup powdered dates or date sugar, sifted through a fine sieve**

**"ESPRESSO" GROUNDS**

**¹⁄₂ tablespoon raisins**

**¹⁄₂ teaspoon raw carob powder**

**FILLING**

**9 large ripe (not overly ripe) bananas**

**¹⁄₄ cup raw agave nectar or sifted powdered dates**

**³⁄₄ cup filtered water (at room temperature)**

**³⁄₄ cup organic, cold-pressed coconut oil or coconut butter**

**CINNAMON DUST**

**¹⁄₂ tablespoon sifted date powder or date sugar**

**¹⁄₂ tablespoon ground cinnamon**

For the crust, in the bowl of a food processor, pulse pecans and powdered dates until the consistency of coarse cornmeal. Do not overprocess. Set aside ¹⁄₂ tablespoon crust mixture to add to the "espresso" grounds. Press half of the remaining crust into the bottom of a 9 x 9-inch baking dish. Place dish in freezer. Set aside remaining half of crust mixture.

For the "espresso" grounds, in the bowl of a food processor, pulse the raisins, carob powder, and reserved ¹⁄₂ tablespoon of "ladyfinger" crust until of uniform consistency. Do not overprocess. Set aside.

For the filling, slice 1¹⁄₂ bananas and set aside. Blend the remaining bananas, in food processor, along with the agave or powdered dates and

water until creamy (scrape down the sides occasionally). While the processor is running, slowly add the coconut oil or coconut butter until incorporated.

For the cinnamon dust, simply mix the ingredients together in a small bowl and set aside.

To assemble, remove the baking dish from the freezer. Pour half of filling on top of crust in baking dish, and smooth with a spatula. Sprinkle half of the "espresso" grounds over filling. Lightly dust with half of the cinnamon-date mixture. (For best results, hold a fine sieve high above dish and tap gently, covering entire surface evenly.) Chill in freezer or refrigerator for 15 to 20 minutes. Remove from freezer. Repeat layers, adding a single layer of sliced bananas after "ladyfinger" crust and before filling. Finishing with remaining "espresso" grounds and cinnamon dust. Chill for 30 minutes. Cut into 3-inch squares and serve.

# creamy carob mousse

**SERVES 2**

*The first time I ate an avocado mousse I was shocked! How could the avocado, which makes my favorite guacamole, also make my most favorite dessert? I can't explain—you must try it for yourself.*

In the bowl of a food processor, use the S blade to blend all the ingredients until creamy. Add water as needed if a lighter consistency is desired. Divide among individual serving dishes and chill until needed.

**2 avocados**

**1 cup raw carob powder**

**1 tablespoon alcohol-free vanilla extract**

**1 teaspoon sea salt**

**5 deglet dates, soaked for 2 to 3 hours**

# appendix

## seeds, beans, and nuts:
## soaking, germinating, and sprouting

Seeds, beans, and nuts are dormant treasure troves of nutrition. Few people know, however, that to unlock them it's not enough to eat them. They need water and time to release their enzyme inhibitors and thus free their full nutritional value.

In addition to being nature's most nutrient-dense food, sprouted seeds and beans are high in fiber that helps clean the colon, and they also help neutralize and remove waste from the body. Some contain substances such as genistein with known anticancer properties.

There are two ways to unlock the nutrients in beans, seeds, and nuts: germinating and sprouting. Germinating is done by merely soaking nuts, seeds, or beans in water for a specific amount of time. The legumes soften and their nutrients are unlocked, but they retain their original shape. Germination is perfect for when you want to make a raw legume edible while keeping most of its original texture.

As an optional additional step, you can sprout your germinated seeds or beans (it's difficult to sprout nuts). Sprouting is germinating taken to the next level. After beans or seeds are germinated, they can be drained and placed in a sprouting container for a specific amount of time. The legume cracks open and a sprout emerges and grows. You're probably familiar with alfalfa sprouts—well, dozens of other beans and seeds can be sprouted and each type of sprout has a unique taste and a subtly different texture. After the legumes sprout, you can eat them immediately or for up to 5 to 6 days. After that, they're likely to become bitter.

Remember to use only raw (dried), preferably organic seeds, beans, and nuts. Roasted seeds or nuts (which are, of course, cooked) will not germinate.

## germinating

Here's a simple way to germinate:

**1.** Rinse your beans, nuts, or seeds, then soak them in purified water for the required germination time (see chart on page 165) in a glass jar or bowl that's covered with cheesecloth or a stocking. They should be soaked at room temperature.

**2.** Afterward, rinse and drain the germinated beans, nuts, or seeds with purified water a couple of times. They are now ready to eat or use in any recipe that calls for them. To sprout the germinated beans or seeds, see below.

## sprouting

Once you've germinated the beans or seeds (see above), you can sprout them if you like. Here's how:

**1.** Place the germinated beans or seeds in a sprouting container, making sure that they are well drained and well ventilated. Cover the container with a fine mesh stocking or cheesecloth to keep bugs out.

**2.** Set the sprouting container on your counter and allow the beans or seeds to sprout for the required sprouting time (see chart on page 165).

**3.** Rinse the sprouted nuts or seeds with purified water a couple of times, and drain well.

**4.** Once they have sprouted, you can eat them right away and for up to 5 to 6 days. After that point, they are likely to be bitter. Store sprouted seeds and beans in an airtight container (not vacuum-sealed) in your refrigerator.

# germination and sprouting chart

| | germination time | sprouting time |
|---|---|---|
| Alfalfa | 8 hours | 2–5 days |
| Almonds* | 8–12 hours | 12 hours |
| Barley | 6–8 hours | 2 days |
| Buckwheat | 6 hours | 2 days |
| Cashews | 2–2½ hours | N/A |
| Chickpeas | 12 hours | 12 hours |
| Kamut | 7 hours | 2–3 days |
| Lentils | 8 hours | 12 hours |
| Mung beans | 1 day | 2–5 days |
| Mustard | 8 hours | 2–7 days |
| Nuts (all others) | 6 hours | N/A |
| Oat groats | 6 hours | 2 days |
| Pumpkin | 8 hours | 1 day |
| Quinoa | 2 hours | 1 day |
| Radish | 8 hours | 2–4 days |
| Red clover | 8 hours | 2–5 days |
| Rye | 8 hours | 3 days |
| Sesame seeds | 8 hours | 1–2 days |
| Spelt | 7 hours | 2 days |
| Sunflower seeds | 2 hours | 2–3 days |
| Walnuts | 4 hours | N/A |
| Wheatberries | 7 hours | 2–2½ days |
| Wild rice | 9 hours | 3 days (sometimes almost 5 days) |

*Almonds are the only nuts that can easily sprout. In fact, they are at their most nutritious when sprouted. After 12 hours of sprouting time, their sprouts are still very small.

# raw resources

At www.carolalt.com, I've put together the kind of one-stop online resource that I wish I'd had when I began learning about raw food. There, you'll find a wealth of information on raw food products and my favorite raw-food Web sites.

You can't always be plugged into the Internet, of course. And sometimes you'll just want to pick up this book and go! So here are some essentials for eating raw—places to buy foods that you can prepare, as well as places where you can go out to eat.

I have not been to every place on this list. This is just a place to start. If you don't like a place, at least question them for recommendations. You should feel comfortable with any place you choose to eat or shop and be sure to look for your *local* health food store!

## natural-food supermarkets

### arizona

#### phoenix

Wild Oats
3933 E. Camelback Rd.
Phoenix, AZ 85018
(602) 954-0584

Whole Foods Market
10810 N. Tatum Blvd.
Phoenix, AZ 85028
(602) 569-7600

Wild Oats
13823 N. Tatum Blvd.
Phoenix, AZ 85032
(602) 953-7546

### scottsdale

Wild Oats
7129 E. Shea Blvd.
Scottsdale, AZ 85254
(480) 905-1441

#### tempe

Whole Foods Market
5120 S. Rural
Tempe, AZ 85282
(480) 456-1400

### tucson

Wild Oats
7133 N. Oracle Rd.
Tucson, AZ 85704
(520) 297-5394

Wild Oats
3360 E. Speedway Blvd.
Tucson, AZ 85716
(520) 795-9844

### arkansas

#### little rock

Wild Oats
10700 N. Rodney Parham
Little Rock, AR 72212
(501) 312-2326

# california

### berkeley

Whole Foods Market
3000 Telegraph Ave.
Berkeley, CA 94705
(510) 649-1333

### beverly hills

Whole Foods Market
239 North Crescent Dr.
Beverly Hills, CA 90210
(310) 274-3360

### brentwood

Whole Foods Market
11737 San Vicente Blvd.
Los Angeles, CA 90049
(310) 826-4433

### campbell

Whole Foods Market
1690 S. Bascom Ave.
Campbell, CA 95008
(408) 371-5000

### chino hills

Henry's Marketplace
3630 Grand Ave.
Chino Hills, CA 91709
(909) 548-0440

### costa mesa

Henry's Marketplace
3030 Harbor Blvd., Suite D
Costa Mesa, CA 92626
(714) 751-6399

### cupertino

Whole Foods Market
20830 Stevens Creek Blvd.
Cupertino, CA 95014
(408) 257-7000

### encinitas

Henry's Marketplace
1327 Encinitas Blvd.
Encinitas, CA 92024
(760) 633-4747

### escondido

Henry's Marketplace
510 W. Thirteenth Ave.
Escondido, CA 92025
(760) 745-2141

### fresno

Whole Foods Market
650 W. Shaw Ave.
Fresno, CA 93711
(559) 241-0300

### glendale

Whole Foods Market
826 North Glendale Ave.
Glendale, CA 91206
(818) 240-9350

Additional Whole Foods
Market planned

### hemet

Henry's Marketplace
1295 S. State St., Suite B
Hemet, CA 92543
(909) 766-6746

### laguna beach

Wild Oats
283 Broadway St.
Laguna Beach, CA 92651
(949) 376-7888

### laguna niguel

Henry's Marketplace
27271 La Paz Rd.
Laguna Niguel, CA 92677
(949) 349-1999

### la jolla

Whole Foods Market
8825 Villa La Jolla Dr.
La Jolla, CA 92037
(858) 642-6700

### la mesa

Henry's Marketplace
4630 Palm Ave.
La Mesa, CA 91941
(619) 460-7722

### lemon grove

Henry's Marketplace
3205 Lemon Grove Ave.
Lemon Grove, CA 91945
(619) 667-8686

### long beach

Wild Oats
6550 E. Pacific Coast Hwy.
Long Beach, CA 90803
(562) 598-8687

### long beach

Whole Foods Market planned

### los angeles

Whole Foods Market
6350 W. Third St.
Los Angeles, CA 90036
(323) 964-6800

### los gatos

Whole Foods Market
15980 Los Gatos Blvd.
Los Gatos, CA 95032
(408) 358-4434

### mill valley

Whole Foods Market
414 Miller Ave.
Mill Valley, CA 94941
(415) 381-1200

### monterey

Whole Foods Market
800 Del Monte Center
Monterey, CA 93940
(831) 333-1600

### northridge

Whole Foods Market
19340 Rinaldi
Northridge, CA 91326
(818) 363-3933

### oakland

Whole Foods Market planned

### palo alto

Whole Foods Market
774 Emerson St.
Palo Alto, CA 94301
(650) 326-8676

### pasadena

Whole Foods Market
3751 E. Foothill Blvd.
Pasadena, CA 91107
(626) 351-5994

Wild Oats
603 S. Lake Ave.
Pasadena, CA 91106
(626) 792-1778

### petaluma

Whole Foods Market
621 E. Washington
Petaluma, CA 94952
(707) 762-9352

### poway

Henry's Marketplace
13536 Poway Rd.
Poway, CA 92064-4725
(858) 486-7851

### redondo beach

Whole Foods Market
405 N. Pacific Coast Hwy.
Redondo Beach, CA 90277
(310) 376-6931

### sacramento

Whole Foods Market
4315 Arden Way
Sacramento, CA 95864
(916) 488-2800

### san diego

Whole Foods Market
711 University Ave.
San Diego, CA 92103
(619) 294-2800

Henry's Marketplace
4439 Genesee Ave.
San Diego, CA 92117
(858) 268-2400

Henry's Marketplace
4175 Park Blvd.
San Diego, CA 92103
(619) 291-8287

Henry's Marketplace
1260 Garnet Ave.
San Diego, CA 92109
(858) 270-8200

Henry's Marketplace
3315 Rosecrans St.
San Diego, CA 92110
(619) 523-3640

Henry's Marketplace
3358 Governor Dr.
San Diego, CA 92122
(858) 457-5006

### san francisco

Whole Foods Market
1765 California St.
San Francisco, CA 94109
(415) 674-0500

Additional Whole Foods
Market planned

### san mateo

Whole Foods Market
1010 Park Place
San Mateo, CA 94403
(650) 358-6900

### san rafael

Whole Foods Market
340 Third St.
San Rafael, CA 94901
(415) 451-6333

### san ramon

Whole Foods Market
100 Sunset Dr.
San Ramon, CA 94583
(925) 355-9000

### santa monica

Whole Foods Market
2201 Wilshire Blvd.
Santa Monica, CA 90403
(310) 315-0662

Wild Oats
1425 Montana Ave.
Santa Monica, CA 90403
(310) 576-4707

Wild Oats
500 Wilshire Blvd.
Santa Monica, CA 90401
(310) 395-4510

### santa rosa

Whole Foods Market
1181 Yulupa Ave.
Santa Rosa, CA 95405
(707) 575-7915

### santee

Henry's Marketplace
9751 Mission Gorge Rd.
Santee, CA 92071
(619) 258-4060

### sebastopol

Whole Foods Market
6910 McKinley St.
Sebastopol, CA 95472
(707) 829-9801

### sherman oaks east

Whole Foods Market
12905 Riverside Dr.
Sherman Oaks, CA 91423
(818) 762-5548

### sherman oaks west

Whole Foods Market
4520 Sepulveda Blvd.
Sherman Oaks, CA 91403
(818) 382-3700

### solana beach

Henry's Marketplace
659 Lomas Santa Fe Dr.
Solana Beach, CA 92075
(858) 350-7900

### thousand oaks

Whole Foods Market
451 Avenida de los Arboles
Thousand Oaks, CA 91360
(805) 492-5340

### torrance

Whole Foods Market
2655 Pacific Coast Hwy.
Torrance, CA 90505
(310) 257-8700

### tustin

Whole Foods Market
14945 Holt Ave.
Tustin, CA 92780
(714) 731-3400

### valencia

Whole Foods Market planned

### walnut creek

Whole Foods Market
1333 E. Newell
Walnut Creek, CA 94596
(925) 274-9700

### west hollywood

Whole Foods Market
7871 W. Santa Monica Blvd.
Los Angeles, CA 90046
(323) 848-4200

### west los angeles

Whole Foods Market
11666 National Blvd.
Los Angeles, CA 90064
(310) 996-8840

### westwood

Whole Foods Market
1050 S. Gayley
Los Angeles, CA 90024
(310) 824-0858

### woodland hills

Whole Foods Market
21347 Ventura Blvd.
Woodland Hills, CA 91364
(818) 610-0000

### yorba linda

Henry's Marketplace
17482 Yorba Linda Blvd.
Yorba Linda, CA 92886
(714) 572-3535

## colorado

### aurora

Wild Oats
12131 E. Iliff Ave.
Aurora, CO 80014
(303) 695-8801

### boulder

Ideal Market
1275 Alpine Ave.
Boulder, CO 80304
(303) 443-1354

Whole Foods Market
Crossroads Common
Shopping Center
2905 Pearl St.
Boulder, CO 80301
(303) 545-6611

Wild Oats
2584 Baseline Rd.
Boulder, CO 80305
(303) 499-7636

Wild Oats
1651 Broadway St.
Boulder, CO 80302
(303) 442-0909

### colorado springs

Wild Oats
5075 N. Academy Blvd.
Colorado Springs, CO 80918
(719) 548-1667

Wild Oats
3180 New Center Point
Colorado Springs, CO 80922
(719) 622-1099

Additional Whole Foods
Market planned

### denver

Wild Oats
900 E. Eleventh Ave.
Denver, CO 80218
(303) 832-7701

Whole Foods Market
2375 E. First Ave.
Denver, CO 80206
(720) 941-4100

Wild Oats
1111 S. Washington St.
Denver, CO 80210
(303) 733-6201

Additional Whole Foods
Market planned

### fort collins

Wild Oats
200 W. Foothills Pkwy.
Ft. Collins, CO 80525
(970) 225-1400

Additional Whole Foods
Market planned

### glendale

Wild Oats
870 S. Colorado Blvd.
Glendale, CO 80246
(303) 691-0101

### golden

Wild Oats
14357 W. Colfax Ave.
Golden, CO 80401
(303) 277-1339

### highlands ranch

Whole Foods Market
9366 South Colorado Blvd.,
Suite B
Highlands Ranch, CO 80126
(303) 470-6003

### littleton

Wild Oats
8194 S. Kipling Pkwy.
Littleton, CO 80127
(720) 214-3174

Wild Oats
5910 S. University Blvd.
Littleton, CO 80121
(303) 798-9699

### westminster

Wild Oats
9229 N. Sheridan Blvd.
Westminster, CO 80031-6530
(303) 650-2333

# connecticut

### greenwich

Whole Foods Market
90 E. Putnam Ave.
Greenwich, CT 06830
(203) 661-0631

### west hartford

Wild Oats
340 N. Main St.
West Hartford, CT 06117
(860) 523-7174

### west hartford

Additional Whole Foods
Market planned

### westport

Wild Oats
399 Post Rd. W.
Westport, CT 06880
(203) 227-6858

# district of columbia

### georgetown

Whole Foods Market
1440 P St. NW
Washington, DC 20005
(202) 332-4300

Whole Foods Market
2323 Wisconsin Ave. NW
Washington, DC 20007
(202) 333-5393

### tenley town

Whole Foods Market
4530 40th St. NW (Tenley Circle)
Washington, DC 20016
(202) 237-5800

# florida

### aventura

Whole Foods Market
21105 Biscayne Blvd.
Aventura, FL 33180
(305) 933-1543

### boca raton

Whole Foods Market
1400 Glades Road, Suite 110
Boca Raton, FL 33431
(561) 447-0000

### coral springs

Whole Foods Market
810 University Dr.
Coral Springs, FL 33071
(954) 753-8000

### ft. lauderdale

Whole Foods Market
2000 North Federal Highway
Ft. Lauderdale, FL 33305
(954) 565-5655

Wild Oats
2501 E. Sunrise Blvd.
Ft. Lauderdale, FL 33304
(954) 566-9333

### melbourne

Wild Oats
1135 W. New Haven Ave.
West Melbourne, FL 32904
(321) 674-5002

### miami beach

Wild Oats
1020 Alton Rd.
Miami Beach, FL 33139
(305) 532-1707

### palm beach gardens

Whole Foods Market planned

### panama city

The Herb Shop
302B West 23rd St.
Panama City, FL 32405
(850) 769-5973

### pinecrest

Wild Oats
11701 S. Dixie Hwy.
Pinecrest, FL 33156
(305) 971- 0900

### plantation

Whole Foods Market
7720 Peters Rd.
Plantation, FL 33324
(954) 236-0600

### sarasota

Whole Foods Market
planned

### west palm beach

Wild Oats
7735 S. Dixie Hwy.
West Palm Beach, FL 33405
(561) 585-8800

### winter park

Whole Foods Market
Winter Park Corners
1989 Aloma Ave.
Winter Park, FL 32792
(407) 673-8788

# georgia

### atlanta

Whole Foods Market
2111 Briarcliff Rd.
Atlanta, GA 30329
(404) 634-7800

Whole Foods Market
650 Ponce de Leon Ave. NE
Atlanta, GA 30308
(404) 853-1681

Whole Foods Market
5930 Roswell Rd.
Atlanta, GA 30328
(404) 236-0810

Additional Whole Foods Market planned

### gwinnett

Harry's Farmer's Market
2025 Satellite Pointe
Duluth, GA 30096
(770) 416-6900

### roswell

Harry's Farmer's Market
1180 Upper Hembree Rd.
Roswell, GA 30076
(770) 664-6300

## illinois

### chicago

Whole Foods Market
30 West Huron
Chicago, IL 60610
(312) 932-9600

Whole Foods Market
3300 N. Ashland
Chicago, IL 60657
(773) 244-4200

Whole Foods Market
1000 West North Ave.
Chicago, IL 60622
(312) 587-0648

Two additional Whole Foods
Markets planned

### deerfield

Whole Foods Market
760 Waukegan Rd.
Deerfield, IL 60015
(847) 444-1900

### evanston

People's Market
1111 Chicago Ave.
Evanston, IL 60202
(847) 475-9492

Whole Foods Market
1640 Chicago Ave.
Evanston, IL 60201
(847) 733-1600

### hinsdale

Wild Oats
500 E. Ogden Ave.
Hinsdale, IL 60521
(630) 986-8500

### palatine

Whole Foods Market
1331 N. Rand Rd.
Palatine, IL 60074
(847) 776-8080

### river forest

Whole Foods Market
7245 Lake St.
River Forest, IL 60305
(708) 366-1045

### wheaton

Whole Foods Market
151 Rice Lake Square
Wheaton, IL 60187
(630) 588-1500

### willowbrook

Whole Foods Market
201 W. Sixty-third St.
Willowbrook, IL 60514
(630) 655-5000

## indiana

### indianapolis

Wild Oats
1300 E. Eighty-sixth St.
Indianapolis, IN 46240
(317) 706-0900

## kansas

### mission

Wild Oats
5101 Johnson Dr.
Mission, KS 66205
(913) 722-4069

### overland park

Whole Foods Market
7401 W. Ninety-first St.
Overland Park, KS 66212
(913) 652-9633

Wild Oats
6621 W. 119th St.
Overland Park, KS 66209
(913) 663-2951

## kentucky

### lexington

Wild Oats
The Mall at Lexington Green
161 Lexington Green Circle
Lexington, KY 40503
(859) 971-8600

### louisville

Wild Oats
4600 Shelbyville Rd.
Louisville, KY 40207
(502) 721-7373

Whole Foods Market planned

## louisiana

### baton rouge

Whole Foods Market planned

### metarie

Whole Foods Market planned

### new orleans

Whole Foods Market
3135 Esplanade
New Orleans, LA 70119
(504) 943-1626

Whole Foods Market
5600 Magazine St.
New Orleans, LA 70115
(504) 899-9119

## maine

### portland

Wild Oats
87 Marginal Way
Portland, ME 04101
(207) 699-2626

## maryland

### annapolis

Whole Foods Market
2504 Solomons Island Rd.
Annapolis, MD 21401
(410) 573-1800

### baltimore

Whole Foods Market
Mount Washington
1330 Smith Ave.
Baltimore, MD 21209
(410) 532-6700

Whole Foods Market
1001 Fleet St., Suite A
Baltimore, MD 21202
(410) 528-1640

### bethesda

Whole Foods Market
5269 River Rd.
Bethesda, MD 20816
(301) 984-4860

### chevy chase

Whole Foods Market planned

### gaithersburg

Whole Foods Market
316 Kentlands Blvd.
Gaithersburg, MD 20878
(301) 258-9500

### rockville

Whole Foods Market
1649 Rockville Pike
Rockville, MD 20852
(301) 984-4880

### silver spring

Whole Foods Market
833 Wayne Ave.
Silver Spring, MD 20910
(301) 608-9373

## massachusetts

### andover

Wild Oats
40 Railroad St.
Andover, MA 01810
(978) 749-6664

### bedford

Whole Foods Market
170 Great Rd.
Bedford, MA 01730
(781) 275-8264

### bellingham

Whole Foods Market
255 Hartford Ave.
Bellingham, MA 02019
(508) 966-3331

### boston

Whole Foods Market
15 Westland Ave.
Boston, MA 02115
(617) 375-1010

Additional Whole Foods
Markets planned

### brighton

Whole Foods Market
15 Washington St.
Brighton, MA 02135
(617) 738-8187

### cambridge

Whole Foods Market
200 Alewife Brook Pkwy.
Cambridge, MA 02138
(617) 491-0040

Whole Foods Market
115 Prospect St.
Cambridge, MA 02139
(617) 492-0070

Whole Foods Market
340 River St.
Cambridge, MA 02139
(617) 876-6990

### framingham

Whole Foods Market
575 Worcester Rd. (Rte. 9)
Framingham, MA 01701
(508) 628-9525

### hadley

Whole Foods Market
Russell St. (Rte. 9)
Hadley, MA 01035
(413) 586-9932

### hingham

Whole Foods Market planned

### medford

Wild Oats
2151 Mystic Valley Pkwy.
Medford, MA 02155
(781) 395-4998

### newton

Whole Foods Market
916 Walnut St.
Newton, MA 02461
(617) 969-1141

### newtonville

Whole Foods Market
647 Washington St.
Newtonville, MA 02458
(617) 965-2070

### saugus

Wild Oats
357 Broadway
Saugus, MA 01906
(781) 233-5341

### wayland

Whole Foods Market
317 Boston Post Rd.
Wayland, MA 01778
(508) 358-7700

### wellesley hills

Whole Foods Market
278 Washington St.
Wellesley Hills, MA 02481
(781) 235-7262

## michigan

### ann arbor

Whole Foods Market
3135 Washtenaw Ave. at
Huron Pkwy.
Ann Arbor, MI 48104
(734) 975-4500

### rochester hills

Whole Foods Market
1404 Walton Blvd.
Rochester Hills, MI 48309
(248) 652-2100

### troy

Whole Foods Market
2880 West Maple
Troy, MI 48084
(248) 649-9600

### west bloomfield

Whole Foods Market
7350 Orchard Lake Rd.
West Bloomfield, MI 48322
(248) 538-4600

## minnesota

### minneapolis

Whole Foods Market
3060 Excelsior Blvd.
Minneapolis, MN 55416
(612) 927-8141

### st. paul

Whole Foods Market
30 S. Fairview
St. Paul, MN 55105
(651) 690-0197

## missouri

### kansas city

Wild Oats
4301 Main St.
Kansas City, MO 64111
(816) 931-1873

### st. louis

Wild Oats
8823 Ladue Rd.
St. Louis, MO 63124
(314) 721-8004

Whole Foods Market
1601 S. Brentwood Blvd.
Brentwood, MO 63144
(314) 968-7744

# nebraska

### omaha

Wild Oats
7831 Dodge St.
Omaha, NE 68114
(402) 397-5047

# nevada

### henderson

Wild Oats
517 N. Stephanie St.
Henderson, NV 89014
(702) 458-9427

### las vegas

Whole Foods Market
8855 W. Charleston Blvd.
Las Vegas, NV 89117
(702) 254-8655

Wild Oats
7250 W. Lake Mead Blvd.
Las Vegas, NV 89128
(702) 942-1500

### reno

Wild Oats
5695 S. Virginia St.
Reno, NV 89502
(775) 829-8666

# new jersey

### edgewater

Whole Foods Market
905 River Rd.
Edgewater, NJ 07020
(201) 941-4000

### madison

Whole Foods Market
222 Main St.
Madison, NJ 07940
(973) 822-8444

### marlton

Whole Foods Market
Greentree Square Shopping
Center
940 Rte. 73 N.
Marlton, NJ 08053
(856) 797-1115

### middletown

Whole Foods Market planned

### millburn

Whole Foods Market
187 Millburn Ave.
Millburn, NJ 07041
(973) 376-4668

### montclair

Whole Foods Market
701 Bloomfield Ave.
Montclair, NJ 07042
(973) 746-5110

### princeton

Wild Oats
255 Nassau St.
Princeton, NJ 08540
(609) 924-4993

Additional Whole Foods
Market planned

### ridgewood

Whole Foods Market
Ridgewood Plaza
44 Godwin Pl.
Ridgewood, NJ 07450
(201) 670-0383

# new mexico

### albuquerque

Wild Oats
6300 San Mateo Blvd. NE,
Suite A
Albuquerque, NM 87109
(505) 823-1933

Whole Foods Market
5815 Wyoming Blvd. NE
Albuquerque, NM 87109
(505) 856-0474

Wild Oats
Indian School Plaza
2103 Carlisle Blvd. NE
Albuquerque, NM 87110
(505) 260-1366

Wild Oats
11015 Menaul Blvd. NE
Albuquerque, NM 87112
(505) 275-6660

### santa fe

Whole Foods Market
753 Cerrillos Rd.
Santa Fe, NM 87501
(505) 992-1700

Wild Oats
1090 S. Saint Francis Dr.
Santa Fe, NM 87505
(505) 983-5333

## new york

### brooklyn

Whole Foods Market planned

### jericho

Whole Foods Market planned

### manhasset

Whole Foods Market
2101 Northern Blvd.
Manhasset, NY 11030
(516) 869-8900

### manhattan

Whole Foods Market
250 Seventh Ave.
New York, NY 10001
(212) 924-5969

Whole Foods Market
10 Columbus Circle
New York, NY 10019
(212) 823-9600

Jubbs Longevity
508 E. 12th St.
New York, NY 10009
(212) 358-8068

Live Live
261 E. 10th St.
New York, NY 10009
(212) 505-5504

Additional Whole Foods
Market planned

### white plains

Whole Foods Market planned

## north carolina

### cary

Whole Foods Market
102B New Waverly Pl.
Cary, NC 27511
(919) 816-8830

### chapel hill

Whole Foods Market
81 S. Elliot
Chapel Hill, NC 27514
(919) 968-1983

### durham

Whole Foods Market
621 Broad St.
Durham, NC 27705
(919) 286-2290

### raleigh

Whole Foods Market
3540 Wade Ave.
Raleigh, NC 27607
(919) 828-5805

### winston-salem

Whole Foods Market
41 Miller St.
Winston-Salem, NC 27104
(336) 722-9233

## ohio

### cincinnati

Wild Oats
2693 Edmondson Rd.
Cincinnati, OH 45209
(513) 531-8015

### cleveland

Wild Oats
27249 Chagrin Blvd.
Cleveland, OH 44122
(216) 464-9403

Additional Whole Foods
Market planned

### upper arlington

Wild Oats
1555 W. Lane Ave.
Upper Arlington, OH 43221
(614) 481-3400

## oklahoma

### tulsa

Wild Oats
1401 E. Forty-first St.
Tulsa, OK 74105
(918) 712-7555

## oregon

### beaverton

Wild Oats
4000 SW 117th Ave.
Beaverton, OR 97005
(503) 646-3824

### bend

Wild Oats
2610 NE Hwy. 20
Bend, OR 97701
(541) 389-0151

### eugene

Wild Oats
2580 Willakenzie Rd.
Eugene, OR 97401
(541) 334-6382

Wild Oats
2489 Willamette St.
Eugene, OR 97405
(541) 345-1014

### gresham

Wild Oats
2077 NE Burnside Rd.
Gresham, OR 97030
(503) 674-2827

### lake oswego

Wild Oats
17711 Jean Way
Lake Oswego, OR 97035
(503) 635-8950

### portland

Whole Foods Market
1210 NW Couch St.
Portland, OR 97209
(503) 525-4343

Wild Oats
3016 SE Division St.
Portland, OR 97202
(503) 233-7374

Wild Oats
3535 NE Fifteenth Ave.
Portland, OR 97212
(503) 288-3414

Wild Oats
6344 SW Capitol Hwy.
Portland, OR 97239
(503) 244-3110

Wild Oats
2825 E. Burnside St.
Portland, OR 97214
(503) 232-6601

# pennsylvania

### devon

Whole Foods Market
821 Lancaster Ave.
Wayne, PA 19087
(610) 688-9400

### jenkintown

Whole Foods Market
1575 Fairway Rd.
Jenkintown, PA 19046
(215) 481-0800

### north wales

Whole Foods Market
1210 Bethlehem Pike
North Wales, PA 19454
(215) 646-6300

### philadelphia

Whole Foods Market
2001 Pennsylvania Ave.
Philadelphia, PA 19130
(215) 557-0015

Whole Foods Market
929 South St.
Philadelphia, PA 19147
(215) 733-9788

### pittsburgh

Whole Foods Market
5880 Centre Ave.
Pittsburgh, PA 15206
(412) 441-7960

### wynnewood

Whole Foods Market
339 E. Lancaster Ave.
Wynnewood, PA 19096
(610) 896-3737

# rhode island

### providence

Whole Foods Market
261 Waterman St.
Providence, RI 02906
(401) 272-1690

Whole Foods Market
University Heights Shopping
Center
601 N. Main St.
Providence, RI 02904
(401) 621-5990

# south carolina

### charleston

Whole Foods Market planned

# tennessee

### franklin

Wild Oats
1735 Galleria, Suite B
Franklin, TN 37067
(615) 778-1910

### memphis

Wild Oats
5022 Poplar Ave.
Memphis, TN 38117
(901) 685-2293

### nashville

Wild Oats
3909 Hillsboro Pike
Nashville, TN 37215
(615) 463-0164

# texas

### arlington

Whole Foods Market
801 E. Lamar
Arlington, TX 76011
(817) 461-9362

### austin

Sun Harvest Farms
2917 W. Anderson Lane
Austin, TX 78757
(512) 451-0669

Sun Harvest Farms
4006 S. Lamar Blvd., Suite 400
Austin, TX 78704
(512) 444-3079

Whole Foods Market
601 N. Lamar, Suite 100
Austin, TX 78703
(512) 476-1206

Whole Foods Market
Gateway (Loop 360 & 183)
9607 Research Blvd.
Austin, TX 78759
(512) 345-5003

Additional Whole Foods Market planned

Quantum Nutritional Labs/Healthline
2000 N. Mays, Suite 126
Round Rock, TX 78664
(800) 370-3447

### corpus christi

Sun Harvest Farms
1440 Airline Rd.
Corpus Christi, TX 78412
(361) 993-2850

### dallas

Whole Foods Market
2218 Lower Greenville Ave.
Dallas, TX 75206
(214) 824-1744

Whole Foods Market
Preston Forest Village
11661 Preston Rd.
Dallas, TX 75230
(214) 361-8887

### el paso

Sun Harvest Farms
6100 N. Mesa St.
El Paso, TX 79912
(915) 833-3380

### highland park

Whole Foods Market
4100 Lomo Alto Dr.
Highland Park, TX 75219
(214) 520-7993

### houston

Whole Foods Market
4004 Bellaire Blvd.
West University Place
Houston, TX 77025
(713) 667-4090

Whole Foods Market
2955 Kirby Dr.
Houston, TX 77098
(713) 520-1937

Whole Foods Market
11145 Westheimer Rd.
Houston, TX 77042
(713) 784-7776

Whole Foods Market
6401 Woodway #149
Houston, TX 77057
(713) 789-4477

### mcallen

Sun Harvest Farms
2008 N. Tenth St.
McAllen, TX 78501
(956) 618-5388

### plano

Whole Foods Market
2201 Preston Rd., Suite C
Plano, TX 75093
(972) 612-6729

### richardson

Whole Foods Market
60 Dal-Rich Village (Coit & Beltline)
Richardson, TX 75080
(972) 699-8075

### san antonio

Sun Harvest Farms
8101 Callaghan Rd.
San Antonio, TX 78230
(210) 979-8121

Whole Foods Market
255 E. Basse Rd., Suite 130
San Antonio, TX 78209
(210) 826-4676

Sun Harvest Farms
2502 Nacogdoches Rd.
San Antonio, TX 78217
(210) 824-7800

Sun Harvest Farms
17700 N. U.S. Hwy. 281,
Suite 200
San Antonio, TX 78232
(210) 499-1446

# utah

### park city

Wild Oats
1748 West Redstone Center
Park City, UT 84098
(435) 575-0200

### salt lake city

Wild Oats
645 E. 400 South
Salt Lake City, UT 84102
(801) 355-7401

Wild Oats
1131 E. Wilmington Ave.
Salt Lake City, UT 84106
(801) 359-7913

# virginia

### alexandria

Whole Foods Market
6548 Little River Turnpike
Alexandria, VA 22312
(703) 914-0040

Additional Whole Foods
Market planned

### arlington

Whole Foods Market
2700 Wilson Blvd.
Arlington, VA 22201
(703) 527-6596

### charlottesville

Whole Foods Market
300 Shoppers World Ct.
Charlottesville, VA 22901
(434) 973-4900

Additional Whole Foods
Market planned

### falls church

Whole Foods Market
7511 Leesburg Pike
Falls Church, VA 22043
(703) 448-1600

### reston

Whole Foods Market
11660 Plaza America Dr.
Reston, VA 20191
(703) 736-0600

### springfield

Whole Foods Market
8402 Old Keene Mill Rd.
Springfield, VA 22152
(703) 644-2500

### vienna

Whole Foods Market
143 Maple Ave. E.
Vienna, VA 22180
(703) 319-2000

# washington

### bellevue

Whole Foods Market planned

### seattle

Whole Foods Market
Roosevelt Square
1026 NE Sixty-fourth St.
Seattle, WA 98115
(206) 985-1500

### vancouver

Wild Oats
8024 E. Mill Plain Blvd.
Vancouver, WA 98664
(360) 695-8878

# wisconsin

### madison

Whole Foods Market
University Plaza
3313 University Ave.
Madison, WI 53705
(608) 233-9566

## CANADA

# british columbia

### vancouver

Capers Community Market
2285 West 4th Ave.
Vancouver, BC, V6K 1N9
(604) 739-6676

Capers Community Market
1675 Robson St.
Vancouver, BC, V6G 1C8
(604) 687-5288

### west vancouver

Capers Community Market
2496 Marine Dr.
West Vancouver, BC,
V7V 1L1
(604) 925-3316

Additional Whole Foods
Market planned

# ontario

### toronto

Whole Foods Market
87 Avenue Road, Box 320
Toronto, ON, M5R 3R9
Canada
(416) 944-0500

# raw restaurants

## alaska

### anchorage

Enzyme Express
1330 E. Huffman Rd.
Anchorage, AK 99515
(907) 345-1330

Jens' Restaurant
Olympic Center
701 W. 36th Ave.
Anchorage, AK 99503
(907) 561-5367
www.jensrestaurant.com
e-mail: jens@alaska.net
*Not entirely raw, and while "this dining spot may be in a mid-town strip mall . . . it is tastefully decorated, featuring Alaskan art, and serves fine food"* (Fodor's Special Recommendation, Fodor's 2003).

## arizona

### patagonia

Tree of Life
771 Harshaw Rd.
Patagonia, AZ 85624
(520) 394-2589
*Patagonia is approximately 1 hour south of Tucson.*

### tempe

Rawesome Café (inside Gentle Strength Co-op)
234 W. University Dr.
Tempe, AZ 85281
(480) 496-5959
www.rawforlife.com
e-mail: info@rawforlife.com
*Call for hours (this cafe is only open a few days a week).*

### tucson

Anjali
330 E. Seventh St.
Tucson, AZ 85733
(520) 623-0913
www.anjali.com
e-mail: info@anjali.com
*A half block west of Fourth Avenue, this is a raw oasis in the middle of an urban desert.*

## california

### berkeley

Raw Energy: Organic Juice Cafe
2050 Addison
Berkeley, CA 94704
(510) 665-9464
*A great place for a quick snack or juice.*

### carmel

Food in the Nude from Cornucopia Community Market
Carmel Rancho Blvd.
Carmel, CA 93923
(831) 620-0520
e-mail: foodinthenude@raw foods.com

### chula vista

Cilantro Live!
315½ Third Ave.
Chula Vista, CA 91910
(619) 827-7401
www.cilantrolive.com

### dunsmuir

Castle Rock Inn
5827 Sacramento Ave.
Dunsmuir, CA 96025
(530) 235-0782
www.castlerockpub.com
e-mail:
bill@castlerockpub.com
*Listen to the river flow outside as you savor American cuisine live food.*

### el cajon

Nature's First Law Raw Superstore
1475 North Cuyamaca St.
El Cajon, CA 92020
(619) 596-7979
www.rawfood.com

### escondido

The Vegetarian
431 W. 13th St.
Escondido, CA 92025
(760) 740-9596
*Not all raw, but all veggie and plenty of raw food on the menu.*

### fairfax

Cafe Sangha
31 Bolinas Ave.
Fairfax, CA 94930
(415) 456-5300
*A new raw-food restaurant nestled in the Bay Area.*

### fountain valley

Au Lac Vegetarian
Restaurant
Mile Square Plaza
16563 Brookhurst
Fountain Valley, CA 92708
(714) 418-0658
www.aulac.com
*Vegetarian with raw options.*

### huntington beach

Good Mood Food Deli Café
5930 Warner Ave.
Huntington Beach, CA 92647
(714) 377-2028
www.goodmoodfood.com
*This café offers Southern California–style raw-food cuisine with an atypical German influence.*

### la jolla

Champions
7523 Fay Ave.
La Jolla, CA
(858) 456-0536

### larkspur

Roxanne's
320 Magnolia Ave.
Larkspur, CA 94939
(415) 924-5004
www.roxraw.com
*Near San Francisco, chef Roxanne Klein presents a first-class culinary experience.*

### middletown

Back to the Garden
21065 Bush St.
Middletown, CA 95461
(707) 987-8303
www.sacreddance.org/garden

### ocean beach

Eatopia
5001 Newport Ave.
Ocean Beach, CA 92107
(619) 224-3237
www.eatopiaexpress.com
e-mail:
eatopia@eatopiaexpress.com
*A small and growing vegan restaurant just north of downtown San Diego with a full juice bar and raw specialties.*

### san francisco

Urban Forage
254 Fillmore St.
San Francisco, CA 94117
(415) 255-6701
www.urbanforage.com
e-mail:
faeries@urbanforage.com

### santa cruz

The 418 Organic Café
418 Front St.
Santa Cruz, CA 95060
(831) 425-LIVE

### santa monica

Juliano's RAW
609 Broadway
Santa Monica, CA 90401
(310) 587-1552
www.rawrestaurant.com
*Juliano is the most colorful, energetic, and controversial raw-food chef out there, known for his book, also called* Raw.

Napoleon
2301 Main St.
Santa Monica, CA 90401
(310) 399-9511
*This is the "other" raw restaurant in Santa Monica and it's cozy and quaint. Just because Juliano's here too, don't miss the amazing and wonderful place where wonderful people gather for delicious food and "good, good, good vibrations."*

# colorado

### durango

Turtle Lake Refuge
826 E. Third Ave.
Durango, CO 81301
(970) 247-8395
*Call ahead to find out when you can stop in for one of their live-food meals.*

# connecticut

## hartford

The Alchemy Juice Bar Cafe
203 New Britain Ave.
Hartford, CT
(860) 246-5700

# district of columbia

Delights of the Garden
2616 Georgia Ave. NW
Washington DC 20001
(202) 319-8747
*Delights of the Garden is a raw-food restaurant located in the heart of the nation's capital.*

# florida

## key west

Dining in the Raw
800 Olivia St.
Key West, FL 33040
(305) 295-2600
*Rita Romano is the author of a book by the same name as her restaurant. This chef, restaurateur, teacher, and dietary consultant was trained at SUNY–Stony Brook, Kushi, and the Hippocrates Institute. Yes, even at the farthest tip of U.S. soil—in Key West—you can find gourmet raw food! It's worth the trip.*

## merritt island

Living Greens
205 McLeod St.
Merritt Island, FL 32953
(321) 454-2268
www.living-greens.com

## miami beach

Food Without Fire
419B Espanola Way
Miami Beach, FL 33139
(305) 674-9960
e-mail:
sunshine_ph@hotmail.com
*I was headed to southern Florida for a week and decided to stop in at this place that is the raw equivalent of a deli—and what I found was not only great food but a banana tiramisu that is to die for! The recipe is on page 160.*

# georgia

## atlanta

Everlasting Life
878 Ralph D. Abernathy Blvd.
Atlanta, GA 30310
(404) 758-1110

## roswell

Sprout Café
1475 Holcolm Bridge Rd., Suite 200
Roswell, GA 30076
(770) 992-9218
www.sproutcafe.com
*This restaurant is operated by the Shinui Retreat in the north suburbs of Atlanta.*

# hawaii

## maui

Westside Natural Foods
193 Lahainaluna
Lahaina, Maui, HI 96761
(808) 667-2855
*Owned by raw foodists, the lunch bar includes an array of raw items beyond the typical, boring salad bar fare.*

# idaho

## ketchum

Akasha Organics
160 North Main St.
Ketchum, ID 83340
(208) 726-4777
e-mail: akasha@svidaho.net
*Part cafe with raw food, part juice bar, part sacred space at the base of the Sun Valley Ski Resort.*

# illinois

## chicago

Karyn's
1901 N. Halsted Ave.
Chicago, IL 60614
(773) 296-6990
www.karynraw.com
*Karyn's Fresh Corner has been around longer than any other raw-food restaurant in the Midwest. The owner, Karyn Calabrese, who is a former model, has been a raw foodist for over twenty-five years. Besides the raw-food restaurant, Karyn and staff operate a full-service spa here too.*

## massachusetts

### beverly

Organic Garden Restaurant
and Juice Bar
294 Cabot St.
Beverly, MA 01915
(978) 922-0004
*The ultimate raw-dining
experience in the Boston area.*

### marblehead

Basil Chef Cuisine
13-R Bessom St.
Marblehead, MA 01945
(781) 864-9250
e-mail: sue@basilchef.com
*Also in the Boston area, this
raw-food restaurant is inside the
Body and Soul health-food store.*

## minnesota

### minneapolis

Ecopolitan
2409 Lyndale Ave. S.
Minneapolis, MN 55405
(612) 87-GREEN (874-7336)
www.ecopolitan.net
e-mail: info@ecopolitan.net
*Completely organic, vegan, and
raw, with an ecological shop
selling natural, nontoxic home
and body products.*

## nevada

### las vegas

Go Raw Café West
2910 Lake East Drive
Las Vegas, NV 89117
(702) 254-5382
www.gorawcafe.com

Go Raw Café East
2381 East Windmill Lane
Las Vegas, NV 89123
(702) 450-9007
www.gorawcafe.com

The Raw Truth Cafe, Healing
Center, and Eco-Shop
3620 East Flamingo Rd.
Las Vegas, NV 89121
(702) 450-9007

## new jersey

### red bank

Down to Earth
7 Broad St.
Red Bank, NJ 07701
(732) 747-4542

## new york

### brooklyn

Green Paradise
609 Vanderbilt Ave.
Brooklyn, NY 11238
(718) 230-5177
e-mail: ckrmr@cs.com
*An organic, raw, vegan
restaurant and juice bar.
Delicious and creative dishes,
many with a Caribbean theme.*

## manhattan

Caravan of Dreams
405 E. Sixth St.
New York, NY 10009
(212) 254-1613
*Organic vegan cuisine with
some excellent raw-food dishes.*

Healthy Pleasures
(Greenwich Village)
93 University Place
New York, NY 10003
(212) 353-3663
*Healthy Pleasures natural foods
stores also offer a cooled and
raw food bar that includes
sashimi, some raw cheeses, and
salads as well as a fresh juice
bar.*

Healthy Pleasures SoHo
489 Broome St.
New York, NY 10013
(212) 431-7434

Jubb's Longevity
508 East Twelfth St.
New York, NY 10009
(888) 420-8270
(212) 358-8068
www.jubbslongevity.com
*Dr. David Jubb's original,
entirely raw take-out style New
York eatery features exquisite
desserts and daily entrées.*

Pure Food and Wine
54 Irving Place
New York, NY 10003
(212) 447-1010
www.purefoodandwine.com
*Celebrity restaurateur Matthew
Kennedy's new raw food
restaurant. I dragged two non-
raw friends kicking and*

*screaming to eat there, and they were amazed by the delicious food.*

Quintessence (Downtown)
263 E. Tenth St.
New York, NY 10009
(646) 654-1823
www.quintessencerestaurant
.com and www.raw-q.com
*Quintessence is a 100 percent raw, organic restaurant servicing the needs of New York City's booming organic raw food movement. If you've been reading this book, you already know that this is my culinary home away from home. When I'm home in New York, I eat here as often as I can. That's often!*

Quintessence
(Upper East Side)
353 E. Seventy-eighth St.
New York, NY 10021
(212) 734-0888

Quintessence
(Upper West Side)
566 Amsterdam Ave.
New York, NY 10024
(212) 501-9700

Spirit New York
530 W. Twenty-seventh St.
New York, NY 10001
(212) 268-9477
info@spiritnewyork.com
*Spirit is a one-of-a-kind hip night spot that intends to touch the whole person and to do so with a style and flair that is second to none. Divided into three distinct areas—Body, Mind, and Soul—the raw food is not found in the Body section of the club (that's for shows with titles like* Rapture *and for dancing). Instead, since feeding the body should also mean feeding the soul, the restaurant is a 180-seat area called Soul. It is both the newest and the largest raw-food restaurant in the Big Apple. Its proprietors intend to open seven such wholistic venues around the globe—an ambitious undertaking. Whether the world is ready for such esprit remains to be seen but surely New York is the place to start.*

Think Liquid Juice Bar
1489 First Ave.
New York, NY 10021
(212) 327-2703
www.thinkliquid.com

# oregon

### ashland

Well Springs Garden Cafe
2253 Highway 99
Ashland, OR 97520
(541) 488-6486
*Raw vegetarian food at the Jackson Hot Springs.*

# pennsylvania

### lansdale

Arnold's Way
319 West Main St.
(Store 4, rear)
Lansdale, PA 19446
(215) 361-0116
www.arnoldsway.com
*A well-established, quaint, delightful restaurant located near Philadelphia offering raw-food meals and juices.*

### malvern

Oasis Living Cuisine
Intersection of Rte. 30 and Rte. 401 in the Great Valley Center
Malvern, PA 19355
(610) 647-9797
www.oasislivingcuisine.com
e-mail:
info@oasislivingcuisine.com
*Despite the name, not all their menu items are living, raw foods. Still, they do make delicious raw things. Breakfast and lunch, closing at 3 P.M.*

# texas

### dallas

Pure
2720 Greenville Ave.
Dallas, TX 75206
(214) 824-7776
www.purerawcafe.com
e-mail:
rawfoodchef@aol.com
*Texas's first raw restaurant. Brand new!*

# washington

### seattle
### (university district)

The Chaco Canyon Cafe
4759 Brooklyn Ave. NE
Seattle, WA 98105
(206) 522-6966
e-mail:
facetphoto@hotmail.com
*Not 100 percent raw but entirely organic, the rotating daily raw menu changes seasonally. The décor is southwestern with beautiful, east-facing windows and both table and counter seating.*

# CANADA

# british columbia

### vancouver

Raw
1849 West 1st Ave.
Vancouver, BC, V6J 5B8
(604) 737-0420
www.rawhealthcafe.com

# manitoba

### winnipeg

The Book Storm/The Raw Experience
107-912 Portage Ave.
Winnipeg, MB, R3G 0P5
(204) 774-1466
e-mail: philar@escape.ca

# ontario

### toronto

Live Health Café
258 Dupont St.
Toronto, ON, M5R 1V7
(416) 515-2002
*This is a cozy space where an innovative menu of fresh, organic, raw vegetarian cuisine is created daily.*

Super Sprouts
205 Spadina Ave.
Toronto, ON, M5T 2C8
(416) 977-7796
www.supersprouts.com
*Super Sprouts is a raw-food resource center located near the exotic fruit shops in Chinatown—not really a restaurant, but you can get ready-to-eat foods to go.*

# quebec

### montréal

Les Vivres
4434 St. Dominique
Montreal, QC, H2T 1R2
(514) 842-3479

# INDONESIA

### ubud, bali

Saru Dori
The Fresh Food Kitchen at Ubud Sari Health Resort
35 Jalan Kajeng
Ubud, Bali, Indonesia
62-361-974-393
*Tropical fruit, organic vegetable dishes, smoothies, quality juices, coconuts, and much more are found on this raw resort's menu. In addition to raw-related health-and-healing programs, colonics, fasting, and a wide range of spa and beauty treatments, you get an exotic, lush, tranquil setting that is sure to change your view of the world and your own life and health.*

# UNITED KINGDOM

### london

VitaOrganic
Wholistic Restaurant, Alternative Cafe and Juice Bar
279c Finchley Rd.
London NW3 6ND
020-7435-2188
*A quaint vegetarian and raw-food restaurant in the heart of London.*

# acknowledgments

I feel so fortunate in my life that whenever I have asked for help I have gotten it. Sometimes we are too proud to ask for help, and sometimes we forget to ask or maybe we are even afraid to ask. Several years back, I was not only not afraid to ask, I did ask, and I got an answer. This book is the fruit of that answer. And I thank God every day for that answer because he lived up to his promise and didn't leave me in my time of need. So, again, thank you, God.

To Bill O'Reilly: From the moment you turned your camera on me many years ago, you have been an inspiration, a confidant, a source of encouragement, and a great friend. Thank you for telling me I had to write a book. Here is that book.

Many people opened their hearts and minds so I could get this down on paper. I want to express my special appreciation and gratitude to Nicholas Gonzalez, MD, in New York City, whose understanding of the science behind the benefits of raw food—and his ability to express that to people—is simply invaluable.

I also need to thank Timothy Brantley, ND. As an instrument of God, he not only changed my life with his thoughts and inspiration, but I have seen him change many lives, every day.

In New York, I have also been fortunate to learn from David Jubb, PhD, of the Longevity Institute and Jubb's Longevity; Danny Hoyt and the whole gang at the Quintessence restaurants; and my fountain of information and reflexologist, Richard Minarek, ND, who also generously provided recipes. Thanks also to David Wolfe of Nature's First Law, San Diego, and to the countless other helpful people too numerous to mention whose knowledge, experience, and expertise have been instructive, illuminating, and inspirational.

Special thanks to Dr. Robert Marshall from Healthline for your generous ideas and proofreading.

For their culinary expertise and recipes, thanks to Kelly Serbonich, executive chef at Hippocrates Health Institute, West Palm Beach, Florida; Juliano of Raw

Juliano in Santa Monica, California; A. J. Hill and Sunshine Phelps at Food Without Fire, Miami Beach, FL; the Lenox Restaurant; and Matthew Johnson at Sushi Samba, in Manhattan.

Thank you to my family—my mom Muriel; brother Tony; sisters Karen and Christine; and niece Katie—for being my guinea pigs and trying new recipes and helping me to remember what it was like when I first decided to go raw—because it was so long ago.

For running out and getting food, taste testing, doing research and being a good sport, thanks to my personal assistant and aspiring fashion designer, Peter Clement.

Thanks to Laura Dail, my agent, and Pam Krauss, Chris Pavone, and especially Adina Steiman at Clarkson Potter, for believing in the message of this book.

And to David Roth, my writer, thank you for clear and compelling writing and sometimes putting up with so much information all at once that I thought you were simply going to explode.

# index

# Introduction to the Second Edition

A recent experience I had in Michigan led me to reflect on the main theme of this book in a new way. I had been invited to speak at a workshop on the Twelve Steps and recovery. My host offered a generous introduction and concluded her remarks by noting that I was the author of *The "Brutal" Path*. We all laughed because it was a genuinely funny moment. It underscored the paradoxical truth that pain and hard work are inevitable on the path to serenity.

This humorous incident, once again, stirred me to ask myself, Why is recovery so hard? One major reason is that recovery is about reclaiming integrity and doing things we initially would rather not. The rewards are not so visible when we begin each new leg of our journey. That's why it's so important to be kind to ourselves along the way. As I thought about the question, I recalled the many therapists who have been genuinely helpful in my life. What they all had in common was a capacity for kindness, compassion, and nurturing coupled with a high degree of personal accountability. They encouraged me not to be so harsh with myself, to view myself with compassion. The tasks of recovery became easier as I listened to their voices.

From my own work as a therapist, I know how hard it is for people to be patient and kind to themselves. One young physician came to our treatment program and used every spare moment of the first three days to completely fill out all the exercises in *The Gentle Path*. His hope was to get done faster. He learned, as we all do, that the process has its own time. Acceptance and surrender are how we become open to healing. I know a group that used *The Gentle Path* for eleven months and only got to the Fourth Step. They were a bit obsessive, perhaps, but they took time for the process. This book aims to help you ease your way through a difficult journey. It does not have to be done fast or perfectly.

In the first edition of *The Gentle Path* we invited readers to send us their reactions to the book and any thoughts on how it might be improved.

1

My vision was that the book would evolve and grow, becoming even more useful over time with the help of its users. The response from around the country has been one of the most gratifying experiences I have had as an author. People have been generous and creative in helping us with this edition.

Thanks to your insightful contributions, we have modified exercises, added new ones, and injected new information. A group guide has been provided as an appendix. We hope you will continue to send us your reactions to this second edition of *The Gentle Path*.

For those who wish to work on some issues more intensively, we have created separate booklets that focus on a particular Step or combination of Steps. We did this for several reasons. Some exercises, such as recording the Personal Craziness Index (PCI), people wanted to do more than once. The second edition provides more writing room, as readers requested, and additional exercises that were extremely helpful but would not fit in the book. We also include a series of meditations and affirmations to support those having a hard time with certain Steps. Most will find that the book is what they want to use. But some may also want to concentrate on a specific Step. The pamphlets will maximize the flexibility of *The Gentle Path* materials for your use. We hope you like what we have done.

No author's work truly stands alone. Many have contributed their insights and expertise to the making of this book. Because of their vital contributions, I especially wish to acknowledge Steven and Toby, Wes and Joanna and The Meadows, Rev. Carolyn Schmidt, Susan F., Gary T., Suzan W., Charlene C., Sheila K., Bobby L., Betty R., Bryan S., Debbie F., and Andrea's Jericho Therapeutic Community.

My thanks also to Ann Marcaccini for her editorial help, Becky Thorvig for keeping things going as we worked on this project, Michael Alvarez and the staff at Del Amo Hospital for their support, and Margaret Marsh and Mark Habrel at CompCare Publishers for believing in the vision.

Patrick J. Carnes
Clinical Director
Sexual Dependency and
  Trauma Recovery Programs
Del Amo Hospital
Torrance, California

# Introduction to the First Edition

This workbook and the accompanying tape set were designed to help people with different types of addictions, including alcoholics, gamblers, compulsive overeaters, and sex addicts, as well as their coaddicted loved ones. Many books exist to help recovering people through the Twelve Steps; some of them even address multiple addictions. This workbook, however, provides a unique set of structured forms and exercises to help you as a recovering person integrate the Twelve Steps into your life.

Gentleness becomes the theme for both the workbook and the audiotape workshop. Addiction by definition possesses a driven quality. Some recovering people try to work the Twelve Steps in the same compulsive manner with which they approached their lives. The spirit of the Twelve Steps is gentleness. The path is a gentle way. Like water wearing down hard rock, consistency and time become allies in creating new channels for one's life.

I hope that the workbook becomes for you a living document that records the basic elements of your story and your recovery. A workbook well used will be filled out completely, frayed at the edges, and have margins crowded with notes. Then, like the Velveteen Rabbit that came alive with use, your "living document" can bring vitality to your program. It can be a way for you to think through issues as you share them with your Twelve Step group, sponsor, therapist, therapy group, or significant others.

Anonymity or confidentiality prevents me from identifying the many people whose suggestions have improved this book of "forms." I am deeply grateful to all of you.

—P.J.C.

# Some Words About Working the Program

Although new members of Twelve Step programs often hear about "working the program," just what that means is often unclear. Each fellowship has its own definition. A bulimic, worried about bingeing, gets one response; an alcoholic, who wants a drink, gets a different one. Even in the same kind of fellowship (such as AA or OA), groups vary according to members' ages, experience, and backgrounds. But some common elements exist that transcend the various fellowships.

Going to Twelve Step meetings is the basic building-block of recovery. Any meeting will help. Usually, a recovering person tries to attend one or two meetings a week, every week. Becoming involved with the life of those meetings provides a solid foundation for recovery. Making a Step presentation in the meetings or taking on a group leadership position, such as treasurer or group representative, are good ways for new members to become involved in the process. The time will come when any meeting will restore the serenity that goes with belonging to the fellowship, but for beginners, as well as experienced members, having a primary group or two anchors them in a program.

Much of working a program, however, goes on outside a meeting. Most recovering people learn about the program from applying program principles to their real-life problems. Members of the group become consultants and teachers as a new member talks about the challenges of early recovery. Those relationships often last a long time. And even if they change, a recovering person learns how to get help from several sources and not to face things alone. Twelve Step fellowships assist people with dependency problems in getting support and effective problem-solving.

Most groups also have a social life outside the meetings. Before or after meetings, people meet for coffee or food. Sometimes favorite restaurants become gathering spots. Some groups have regular breakfasts or lunches where people gather as sort of a "second" group meeting for extra support. Some groups have retreats together to intensify work on the program. While these are not part of the meeting, they are essential to program life. To regard them as an option for which one does not have time is to miss out on an important part of developing a program for oneself: building a support network.

One major obstacle you may need to overcome as a new member is a reluctance to use the telephone. To feel comfortable only when talking about serious issues face to face limits your ability to use your consultants. Addicted people are not good at asking for help in general, and they will resist using the phone even at the most critical times. Thus, they stay in their isolation. Using the phone can become a habit. At first it serves as a crisis hotline. As recovery progresses, it becomes a tool for maintaining and deepening intimacy. Some program veterans hold on to their phone phobias and still put together successful recoveries. They are rare, however. Many groups urge newcomers to get a phone list and make "practice" calls from the start.

A key figure in developing a program is your sponsor. The Twelve Steps in many ways are a demanding discipline. At whatever stage of recovery, early as well as advanced, new challenges emerge constantly in applying the Steps. Recovering people select a sponsor (sometimes two) to serve as a principal guide and witness. In early recovery, contact with a sponsor is often daily—and at times hourly. The sponsor does not have to be much more "expert" than you. Your sponsor is simply someone who

- Agrees to be your sponsor
- Knows your whole story
- Can hold you accountable for how you work your program
- Keeps the focus on how the Steps apply to your life
- Can be honest with you
- Will support you

Sometimes sponsorship evolves into friendship, but the sponsor's chief goal is to help you understand your story. Sponsors also enhance their recoveries by helping you.

Twelve Step fellowships exist to help people stop self-destructive behavior over which they are powerless. Central to stopping the behavior is defining sobriety. Sometimes that is difficult to do. What is a slip for a codependent or a compulsive eater? Does sobriety mean just abstinence for the alcoholic, or is other behavior to be avoided as well? Most recovering people find that their understanding of "sobriety" evolves over time—and that it goes beyond just stopping self-destructive behavior. It also means embracing new behaviors. Later in this workbook you will have a chance to examine your definition of sobriety. At the outset, however, you will need to talk with your sponsor and your group about what you will not do. You may be powerless over your addiction, but you are responsible for your recovery.

Many people find initiating a recovery program extremely difficult. In earlier times, the only solution when things got rough was to attend more meetings. Fortunately, professional therapists and treatment facilities now support the recovery process for the many forms of addictive illness. They have become extended partners to the fellowship. When you feel discouraged, read the "Big Book" of Alcoholics Anonymous—the original fellowship — especially Chapters Five and Six. Composed in the days when professional support was unavailable and even hostile to Twelve Step groups, it serves as inspiration to all who wish to transform their lives.

The Twelve Steps form a process that promotes two qualities in its membership: honesty and spirituality. Starting with the first admission of powerlessness, the Steps demand a high level of accountability to oneself and others. Only one way exists to maintain that level of integrity: a committed spirituality. The fellowship becomes a community that supports this process. The program, however, is not abstract, but very concrete. You "work" your program whenever you

- Make a call for support
- Do a daily meditation of the program
- Admit your powerlessness
- Are honest about your mistakes and shortcomings
- Have a spiritual awareness
- Support another program person

- Actively work on a Step
- Work for balance in your life
- Focus on today
- Take responsibility for your choices, feelings, and actions
- Do something to mend harm you caused
- Attend a meeting
- Give a meeting
- Maintain a defined sobriety

Addicts and coaddicts live in the extremes. No middle ground exists. You, as an addict, are like a light switch that is either totally on or totally off. Life, however, requires a rheostat, a switch mechanism in which there are various degrees of middle ground. Mental health involves a disciplined balance that relies on self-limits and boundaries. Nowhere is that more evident than in the two core issues that all addicts (including coaddicts) face: intimacy and dependency.

The most obvious extreme is dependency on a mood-altering drug or experience (like sex, gambling, or eating) to cope with life. The chemical or experience becomes the trusted source of nurturing or a way to avoid pain or anxiety. All else is sacrificed or compromised. Workaholism, compulsive spending, high-risk experiences (skydiving or racing) simply fill out the range of options to lose oneself.

In the grip of addiction or obsessive behavior, life becomes chaotic and crisis-filled. Addicts and coaddicts live in excess and on the edge. Because they do not complete things, they have much unfinished business. They lack boundaries, so they often do not use good judgment. Others see them as irresponsible and lacking in common sense.

The opposite excessive extreme is grounded in overcontrol. Sexual obsession, for example, can be expressed as either sexual addiction or compulsive abstinence. Many adult children of alcoholics who become compulsive nondrinkers are as obsessed with alcohol as their alcoholic parent(s). An anorexic and a compulsive overeater are both obsessed with food. Overcontrol may be reflected in behaviors such as compulsive dieting and saving, extreme religiosity, phobic responses, panic attacks, and procrastination.

For those with a strong need to control people, events, or their emotions, life becomes rigid, empty, and sterile. Risks are to be avoided at all costs. The fear of beginning new projects or experimenting with new behaviors is sustained by harsh judgmental attitudes and perfectionism. Living in deprivation may seem better than being out of control. But it is still an obsessive lifestyle that leads to loss of self. Recovering people can fall into a real trap if they switch from one extreme to the other and believe that the shift equals true change.

| Out of Control | Overcontrol |
| --- | --- |
| Alcoholism | Compulsive nondrinking |
| Sex addiction | Compulsive nonsexuality |
| Compulsive eating | Anorexia |
| Compulsive gambling | Extreme religiosity |
| High-risk experiences | Phobic responses |
| Workaholism | Procrastination |
| Compulsive spending | Compulsive saving |

| Life Becomes | Life Becomes |
| --- | --- |
| Chaotic | Rigid |
| Living on the edge | Risk avoidant |
| Crisis-filled | Empty |
| Unfinished | Fear of beginning |
| No common sense | Judgmental |
| Irresponsible | Perfection |
| Excess | Deprivation |

When some of these obsessive behaviors mix, life becomes even more complex. Consider this couple: He is a sex addict and an alcoholic, and she is a compulsive overeater. She attempts to control his addiction by throwing out his *Playboys* and his booze. He monitors her eating and criticizes her weight. They are both codependent. Each is obsessed with what the other is doing, each believing that he or she has the power to change the other. As his sex addiction becomes more out of control (although he believes he can control it), she becomes more nonsexual, acting as if she has the power to balance the equation. Even her excessive weight becomes a way for her to exert power by making her sexually unattractive. The reality is they are both powerless in some ways they have not acknowledged.

Variations on this theme plague couples and families in which addiction thrives. A person can even live in simultaneous internal extremes. For example, think of the bulimic who both binges (overeats) and purges (vomits). Only one way exists for people to fight living in such addictive extremes: to admit to the reality of their powerlessness.

To accomplish that task, another issue needs to be faced: intimacy. Addicts and coaddicts seek closeness, nurturing, and love. In many ways addiction derives its compelling force because of a failure of intimacy. Addictive (again including coaddictive) obsession replaces human bonding and caring.

With no emotional rheostat, you can live an isolated, lonely existence in which you build walls around yourself, deny your own needs, and share nothing of yourself. Or, you flip to an emotionally enmeshed existence in which you are so overinvolved you feel trapped and smothered. You concentrate on meeting the needs of another person and take responsibility for that person's behavior. No boundaries exist and consequently no privacy exists. Again, a pattern of living in the extremes emerges.

| Isolated | Enmeshed |
|:---:|:---:|
| Denial of needs | Needs of others are priority |
| Lonely | Smothered |
| No sharing | No privacy |
| Alienated from others | Responsible for others |
| Extreme boundaries | No boundaries |

Add out of control with isolated—that's one extreme and you get off center; add overcontrol with enmeshed and you get off center in another way.

## Addiction/Coaddiction

**Extreme Living**

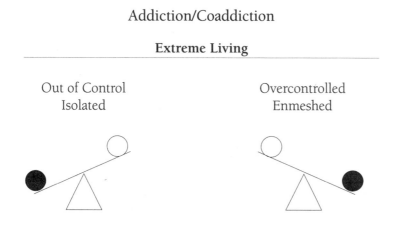

Out of Control
Isolated

Overcontrolled
Enmeshed

## Recovery

**Centered Living**

Balance, Focus, Responsibility for Self

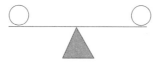

The Twelve Steps offer you a path out of extreme living. Three themes remain constant throughout the Twelve Step process: balance, focus, and responsibility for self.

**Balance:** to avoid either-or extremes

**Focus:** to live in the present—a day at a time—not in the future or the past

**Responsibility for self:** to live within your own human limits

With these three themes as a basis for living your life, recovery becomes possible.

---

### ❧ My Recovery Themes ❧

Balance

Focus

Responsibility for self

---

Before thoroughly pursuing your path, you need to secure guides to support you and help you find your way. Usually this starts with your sponsor. A sponsor is a person who works with you to help you understand the program you undertake. Other members of your Twelve Step group, or, if you are in therapy, your therapist, can also serve as guides. Record on the next page who your guides will be.

This workbook concludes with a set of suggested readings. The workbook also provides a format to supplement your guides, your reading, and if you have the companion tapes, your listening. A thoughtful approach on your part will enhance the workbook. Your guides will also make suggestions, especially about reading material appropriate to your program.

## ❧ My Guides Will Be ❧

### Sponsor

---

### Others

---

---

---

# Step One

## We admitted we were powerless over alcohol— that our lives had become unmanageable.

In every culture of the world, human beings have created myths and legends to give their lives meaning and to describe the significant events and relationships that shape their experiences. In *The Hero with a Thousand Faces*, Joseph Campbell traced the origin of humanity's most universal story: the hero's journey. After studying the literature of civilizations past and present, Campbell concluded that these myths expressed important truths about the human condition. The struggles to break free from rigid, soul-stifling rules, develop a relationship with God, and express one's unique identity are universal.

The archetypes described in these myths also surface in dreams. According to Carl Jung, these archetypes represent different aspects of the human mind; our personalities divide themselves into a variety of characters who play out the inner dramas of our lives. That is why we feel a sense of recognition and identification with them. To be healthy, we need to understand the lessons they can teach us about ourselves.

One of the most important archetypes is that of the hero who overcomes adversity and becomes transformed as a result. Heroes discover, in their limitations, dramatic and unforeseen strengths. All of us have a hero within. Recovering people who have been in recovery for some time almost always marvel at the expanded awareness and renewed capabilities their suffering has brought. They have walked the ancient path of the hero.

In every sense, you are beginning the hero's journey. Most heroes, whether it be Luke Skywalker, Bilbo Baggins, or Hamlet, begin reluctantly. Forces beyond their control propel them past the busyness of their lives and into personal change and renewal. In *Star Wars IV: A New Hope*, Luke Skywalker is on a quest to destroy Darth Vader's evil empire. But Yoda, a wise teacher and spiritual guide, tells Luke of a more important struggle within. A major part of Luke's battle for peace and justice involves confronting his own shadow or dark side. "You will face only what you bring with you," Yoda says. Luke's first teacher, Obe Wan Kanobe, gave another warning: "Things are not what they seem. Your eyes can deceive you. Don't trust them. Reach out with your feelings."

If you are like most addicts, you are unaware of parts of yourself, including your feelings. Without that self-knowledge, you misperceive your own reality. The First Step is designed to give you what you need to know for your journey.

The First Step requires an admission of powerlessness over living in the extremes. As part of this Step, you assemble evidence to document both powerlessness and unmanageability in your life. This is the beginning of understanding the story of your illness. Clearly specifying the history becomes essential to the unfolding of the story. The following exercises will help you in documenting your history.

**Affirmations** — Addicts and coaddicts have been negatively programmed. The experience of their illness only confirmed the damaging messages from their childhood. A list of affirmations is provided to help you reprogram. Use them daily and as you need them.

**Consequences Inventory** — You may have grown so used to life as an addict, or life with an addict, that what is normal becomes obscure. The Consequences Inventory helps to identify behaviors, attitudes, feelings, and results that indicate that life is unmanageable.

**Family Tree and Addiction** — Most addicts have other addicts and coaddicts in their families. By thinking through your family tree, some patterns may emerge that will show how some part of your powerlessness started within your family.

**Addiction History** — Addicts and coaddicts frequently have other addictions that affect their powerlessness. One example is that of the addict whose alcoholic behavior increases his sexual acting out. Another example is the codependent whose excessive weight gain from compulsive overeating increases feelings of unworthiness.

**Abuse Checklist** — Sexual, physical, and emotional abuse are common in addictive families. Children are powerless over the abuse they receive from the adults in their lives. The abuse damaged them in fundamental ways that serve as catalysts to their becoming addicted and coaddicted.

**Step One for Addicts** — Once you have documented your history in the above exercises, you'll be ready to start working and reflecting on your First Step. You'll begin to carefully document the powerlessness and unmanageability in your own life.

**Step One for Coaddicts** — You'll specify the type of addiction to which you are coaddicted and document your powerlessness and unmanageability.

*Note for all addicts:* A high probability exists that you are coaddicted as well. At some point you may wish to return and do a First Step on your coaddiction.

**Sharing Your First Step** — Part of taking the First Step is sharing what you've learned about your story with your guides and others in the program. Remember, the answers may not come easily as you complete the exercise. When you feel stuck, get your guides to help you!

# Affirmations

One cost of addiction is loss of faith in abilities. We can learn to reprogram ourselves with positive, healthy messages.

A list of suggested affirmations follows. Each affirmation is written in the present—as if you are already accomplishing it. It may not be a reality for you today. You need to "act as if." It may be difficult, but think of it as planting a garden with possibilities that will blossom into wonderful realities.

Select from the list the affirmations that have meaning for you. Add some of your own. Tape the list of affirmations on your mirror and repeat them while you are shaving or putting on your makeup. Keep a copy in the car to repeat while commuting, or record these comforting words on a tape and listen to them before you go to bed.

& Today I accept that the life I have known is over.

& I am entering a new and blessed phase of my time here.

& I accept pain as my teacher and problems as the key to a new existence for me.

&#10052; I seek guides in my life and understand that they may be different than I anticipate.

&#10052; I accept the messages surrounding me. Negativity is replaced with positive acceptance.

&#10052; I realize that I have had a hard life and that I deserve better.

&#10052; I let the Spirit melt the hardness of my heart.

&#10052; I comfort and nurture myself. As part of the surren der of my pride I will let others give to me as an act of faith in my value as a person.

&#10052; I accept my illness as part of the trauma of this cul ture and my family.

&#10052; I appreciate that in the chaos of the now, my instinct and beliefs may work against me. My recovering friends help me sort out healthy instincts and beliefs from unhealthy ones.

&#10052; Time is transforming my loneliness into solitude, my suffering into meaning, and relationships into intimacy.

&#10052; I do not blame or search for fault. It is not who, but how, and what happened.

&#10052; I commit to reality at all costs knowing that is where I will find ultimate serenity.

&#10052; I accept that life is difficult and that leaning into the struggle adds to my balance.

Create affirmations that are meaningful to you:

_____

_____

_____

# Consequences Inventory

The movie *Mask* is about a boy whose face is grossly disfigured from an illness. The story deals with the prejudice of other people and what others learn from the boy's courage. In one scene, the boy and his mother go into a typical carnival fun house and look into the distorted mirrors. Instead of reflecting his grossly misshapen face, the warped mirror reveals the image of a normal boy. He calls his mother over and they stare at what he would look like without his disease.

Addiction is like living in a fun house. The insanity and unmanageability of addiction and codependency look normal to those who can see themselves only through the distorted lens of dysfunctional behavior and its consequences. The warped mirrors of the addict or coaddict make the bizarre look normal. The following exercises are designed to break the mirrors that distort our reality.

Check each of the following that you have experienced:

## Emotional Consequences

❏    1. Attempted suicide

❏    2. Suicidal thoughts or feelings

❏    3. Homicidal thoughts or feelings

❏    4. Feelings of extreme hopelessness or despair

❏    5. Failed efforts to control the addiction or the addict

❏    6. Feeling like two people—living a public and a secret life

❏    7. Emotional instability (depression, paranoia, fear of going insane)

❏    8. Loss of touch with reality

❏    9. Loss of self-esteem

❑ 10. Loss of life goals

❑ 11. Acting against your own values and beliefs

❑ 12. Strong feelings of guilt and shame

❑ 13. Strong feelings of isolation and loneliness

❑ 14. Strong fears about your future

❑ 15. Emotional exhaustion

❑ 16. Other emotional consequences; specify:

_____

_____

_____

_____

## Physical Consequences

❑ 1. Continuation of addictive behavior despite the risk to your health

❑ 2. Extreme weight loss or gain

❑ 3. Physical problems (e.g., ulcers, high blood pressure)

❑ 4. Physical injury or abuse by others

❑ 5. Involvement in potentially abusive or dangerous situations

❑ 6. Vehicle accidents (e.g., automobile, motorcycle, bicycle)

❑ 7. Self-abuse or injury (e.g., cutting, burning, bruising)

❑ 8. Sleep disturbances (e.g., not enough sleep, too much sleep)

❑ 9. Physical exhaustion

❑  10.  Other physical consequences, specific to your addiction or codependency (e.g., blackouts, venereal disease, AIDS, bleeding from the throat or nose, vulnerability to disease)

_____

_____

_____

_____

## Spiritual Consequences

❑  1.  Strong feelings of spiritual emptiness

❑  2.  Feeling disconnected from yourself and the world

❑  3.  Feeling abandoned by God or Higher Power

❑  4.  Anger at your Higher Power or God

❑  5.  Loss of faith in anything spiritual

❑  6.  Other spiritual consequences; specify:

_____

_____

_____

_____

## Family and Partnership Consequences

❑  1.  Risking the loss of partner or spouse

❑  2.  Loss of partner or spouse

❑  3.  Increase in marital or relationship problems

❑  4.  Jeopardizing the well-being of your family

❑  5.  Loss of your family's or partner's respect

❏ 6. Increase in problems with your children

❏ 7. Loss of your family of origin

❏ 8. Other family or partnership consequences;
specify:

_____

_____

_____

_____

## Career and Educational Consequences

❏ 1. Decrease in productivity at work

❏ 2. Demotion at work

❏ 3. Loss of co-workers' respect

❏ 4. Loss of the opportunity to work in the career of your choice

❏ 5. Failing grades in school

❏ 6. Loss of educational opportunities

❏ 7. Loss of business

❏ 8. Forced to change careers

❏ 9. Not working to capability (underemployed)

❏ 10. Termination from job

❏ 11. Other career or educational consequences; specify:

_____

_____

_____

_____

## Other Consequences

☐    1. Loss of important friendships

☐    2. Loss of interest in hobbies or activities

☐    3. Few friends who don't participate in your addiction or your partner's addiction

☐    4. Financial problems

☐    5. Illegal activities (arrests or near-arrests)

☐    6. Court or legal involvement

☐    7. Lawsuits

☐    8. Prison or workhouse

☐    9. Stealing or embezzling to support behavior

☐  10. Other consequences; specify:

_____

_____

_____

_____

# Family Tree and Addiction

Most addicts and coaddicts come from families in which addiction or compulsive behavior was present. We learned to cope with addictive or codependent behavior by denying our feelings, wants, and needs. To help understand your powerlessness over the sources of your shame, diagram your family of origin back three generations. After entering each person's name, record any compulsive or addictive characteristics on the line below the person's name. If you are unsure, but you have a good guess about a person, simply write in the information and circle it.

## Compulsive or Addictive Characteristics

1.  alcoholic

2.  compulsive gambler

3.  anorexic/bulimic

4.  compulsive overeater

5.  sex addict

6.  victim of child abuse

7.  perpetrator of child abuse

8.  mental health problem

9.  other compulsive or addictive behavior such as overeating, working, spending, or extreme religiosity (please label)

10. coaddict

# Family Tree and Addiction Chart

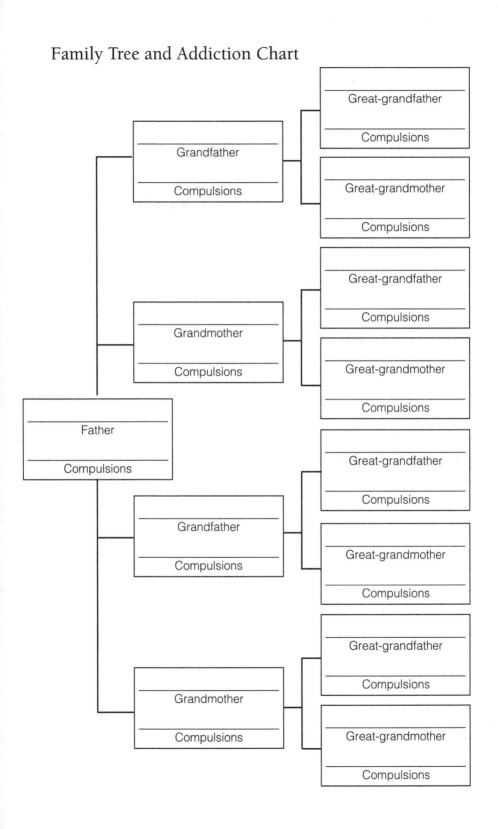

# Family Tree and Addiction Chart

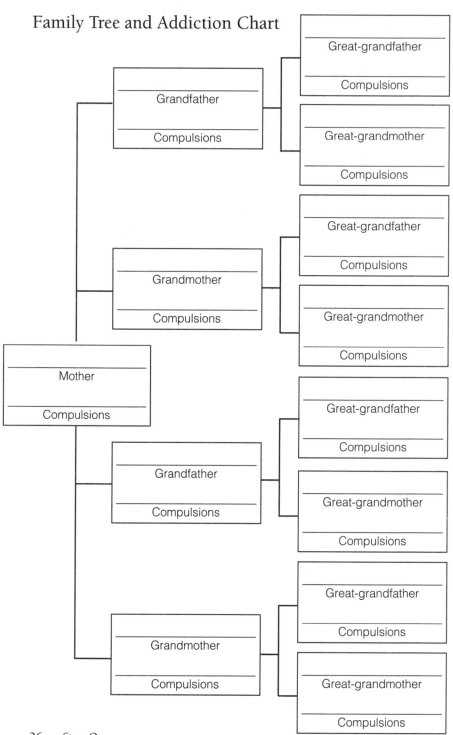

Now list any other relatives (brothers, sisters, uncles, aunts, or cousins) who fit one of the ten categories.

Example: Fred Smith, uncle, alcoholic, sex addict.

1. _____

2. _____

3. _____

4. _____

5. _____

6. _____

7. _____

8. _____

9. _____

10. _____

Are there patterns of addiction in your family? Given the role of addiction in your family, what reflections do you now have about your own powerlessness? Can you see ways in which your addictive behavior was learned, or ways in which your behavior was a form of coping with an unhealthy family environment?

Record your reflections here:

_____

_____

_____

_____

_____

_____

# Addiction History

Addictions and obsessions migrate. Witness the alcoholic who gets sober and then starts acting out sexually. His sexual behavior, which was already out of control, escalates dramatically to fill the obsessive void created when he stopped drinking. Our addictions and obsessions can also support one another. The compulsive gambler/sex addict who goes to Las Vegas for a multiple binge is a good example. Because addictions are "cunning and baffling," the type of addiction may shift from one extreme to another; for example, the compulsive overeater may become anorexic. Addictions and compulsions may become part of the family system. Consider the alcoholic whose codependent obsession with his wife's compulsive eating is an excuse for him to drink.

As part of the First Step, it helps to chronicle how various addictions or self-abusive behaviors have affected one another. Review the following categories of addictive or "unstoppable" behaviors. Simply write examples of how other out-of-control behaviors affected the development of your addiction or coaddiction during each age category. The notes can be short and descriptive.

Example: Compulsively masturbating at age 6 in order to sleep—was worse when Dad was drunk and violent—using sex to deal with my codependent fear.

Another example: My weight was heaviest at 29 when I was trying to control my spouse's addiction.

| Behavior | Age 0–10 | Age 11–18 | Age 19–25 | Age 26–40 | Age 41+ |
|----------|----------|-----------|-----------|-----------|---------|
| Eating   |          |           |           |           |         |

| Behavior | Age 0–10 | Age 11–18 | Age 19–25 | Age 26–40 | Age 41+ |
|----------|----------|-----------|-----------|-----------|---------|
| Alcohol  |          |           |           |           |         |

| Behavior | Age 0–10 | Age 11–18 | Age 19–25 | Age 26–40 | Age 41+ |
|---|---|---|---|---|---|
| Sexuality | | | | | |

| Behavior | Age 0–10 | Age 11–18 | Age 19–25 | Age 26–40 | Age 41+ |
|----------|----------|-----------|-----------|-----------|---------|
| Gambling |          |           |           |           |         |

| Behavior | Age 0–10 | Age 11–18 | Age 19–25 | Age 26–40 | Age 41+ |
|----------|----------|-----------|-----------|-----------|---------|
| Coaddiction | | | | | |

| Behavior | Age 0–10 | Age 11–18 | Age 19–25 | Age 26–40 | Age 41+ |
|---|---|---|---|---|---|
| Other examples of compulsive behavior (give label—for example, shoplifting, spending, smoking, working, dangerous or high-risk behaviors) | | | | | |

Now that you have completed your addiction history, think about how your addictions and codependency affected one another. How does looking at the patterns of "extreme" living help you in looking at your First Step?

Record your reflections here:

_____

_____

_____

_____

_____

_____

_____

_____

_____

_____

_____

_____

_____

_____

_____

_____

_____

_____

_____

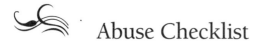 Abuse Checklist

Addiction studies show a high correlation between childhood emotional, physical, and sexual abuse and subsequent addiction. The following checklist and worksheet will help you assess the extent to which you were abused in your own childhood. To cope with your own abuse, you may have minimized the impact the abuse had on your life. Now is the time to recognize the abuse for what it was. Know that it was not your fault, and recognize your powerlessness over it.

Read over each of the three categories of abuse (emotional, physical, and sexual). Fill in the information in the spaces next to the items that apply to you. For each type of abuse, record the information to the best of your memory.

These are powerful memories. In thinking about these acts, be aware that an absence of feelings is a sign that you may be avoiding the work that needs to go into this Step.

| | |
|---|---|
| Age | How old were you when the abuse started? |
| Abusing persons | Who abused you? Father, stepfather, mother, stepmother, adult relative, adult friend, adult neighbor, neighborhood children, professional person, brother or sister, or stranger? |
| Frequency | How often did it happen? Daily, two to three times a week, weekly, monthly? You may use the following scale: 1 = one time; 2 = seldom; 3 = periodically; 4 = often; and 5 = very often. |

| Form of Abuse | Age | Frequency | Abusing Person |
|---|---|---|---|
| Emotional Abuse | | | |
| Example: Neglect | 3 | 5 | grandparent, father |
| Neglect (ie., significant persons are emotionally unavailable; emotional or physical care is inadequate) | | | |
| Harassment or malicious tricks | | | |
| Being screamed at or shouted at | | | |
| Unfair punishments | | | |
| Cruel or degrading tasks | | | |
| Cruel confinement (e.g., being locked in closet; excessive grounding for long periods) | | | |
| Abandonment (e.g., lack of supervision, lack of security, being left or deserted, death or divorce removing primary care-givers) *(Continued)* | | | |

| Form of Abuse | Age | Frequency | Abusing Person |
|---|---|---|---|
| Touch deprivation | | | |
| Overly strict dress codes | | | |
| No privacy | | | |
| Having to hide injuries or wounds from others | | | |
| Forced to keep secrets | | | |
| Having to take on adult responsibilities as a child | | | |
| Having to watch beating of other family members | | | |
| Being caught in the middle of parents' fights | | | |
| Being blamed for family problems | | | |
| Other forms of emotional abuse | | | |

| Form of Abuse | Age | Frequency | Abusing Person |
|---|---|---|---|
| **Physical Abuse** | | | |
| Example: Shoving | 8, 18–30 | 5 | |
| Mother, stepfather, spouse | | | |
| Shoving | | | |
| Slapping or hitting | | | |
| Scratches or bruises | | | |
| Burns | | | |
| Cuts or wounds | | | |
| Broken bones or fractures | | | |
| Damage to internal organs | | | |
| Permanent injury | | | |

*(Continued)*

| Form of Abuse | Age | Frequency | Abusing Person |
|---|---|---|---|
| Beatings or whippings | | | |
| Inadequate medical attention | | | |
| Pulling and grabbing of hair, ears, etc. | | | |
| Inadequate food or nutrition | | | |
| Other forms of physical abuse | | | |

| Form of Abuse | Age | Frequency | Abusing Person |
|---|---|---|---|
| **Sexual Abuse** | | | |
| Example:<br>Flirtatious and<br>suggestive language | 6, 12–17 | 4 | Stranger, adult neighbor |
| Propositioning | | | |
| Inappropriate holding, kissing | | | |
| Sexual fondling | | | |
| Masturbation | | | |
| Oral sex | | | |
| Forced sexual activity | | | |
| Household voyeurism<br>(inappropriate household<br>nudity, etc.) | | | |
| Sexual hugs | | | |
| Jokes about your body | | | |

*(Continued)*

| Form of Abuse | Age | Frequency | Abusing Person |
|---|---|---|---|
| Use of sexualizing language | | | |
| Penetration with objects | | | |
| Bestiality (forced sex with animals) | | | |
| Criticism of your physical or sexual development | | | |
| Another's preoccupation with your sexual development | | | |
| Other forms of sexual abuse | | | |

A way to view trauma is to look at two factors. First is how significant the impact was. Second is how often the abuse happened. So, for example, you could have something happen just a few times, but it may have a very harmful effect on you. Similarly, something done that in itself is not that harmful but is done repeatedly may cause severe stress. Look at Figure 1 to see the relationship between frequency and impact of abuse.

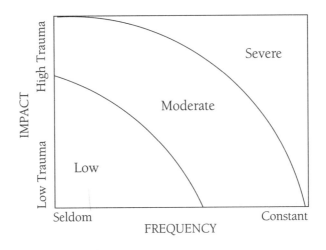

Figure 1  Impact of Abuse

For example, if you experienced touch deprivation occasionally, you might not consider the deprivation very important. But if you were deprived constantly, you might view your situation quite differently. It is not just the quantity that is important, but how you experienced the abuse that is important.

For many of us, denying the pain and reality of what was done to us has been a source of our insanity. Accepting our powerlessness is not saying that it was okay; it is recognizing, maybe for the first time, that the abuse was not okay. Until we can accept the fear, anger, and sadness, we cannot grieve. It is our grieving that helps us to accept our powerlessness.

How has the abuse you received as a child affected you? How do you feel in reflecting on these events? What has been the impact on your addictive or coaddictive behavior? Record your answers on the next page.

# Gentleness Break

You have just completed a significant piece of work. Congratulations! Before you continue with the First Step exercise, stop and reward yourself. Choose one or more of the following activities to be gentle with yourself. If none of these appeals to you, find one of your own. If you feel compelled to keep on working, remember that you can become compulsive about the workbook, too.

Pet a warm puppy.

Play with a child.

Enjoy a long nap.

Make a cup of tea.

Walk with a friend.

Ask for a hug.

Do something not useful but fun.

Sit by a lake or a stream.

Work in a garden.

Meditate.

Listen to favorite music.

Talk with a friend.

Read a novel.

Watch the sun set.

Sit with a teddy bear.

Ask someone to nurture you.

# Step One for Addicts

> We admit we are powerless over
>
> _____
>
> (insert alcohol or sex, etc.)
> and that our lives have become unmanageable.

Acceptance of the First Step paves the way to recovery. As you grow to understand your own powerlessness and how unmanageable your life became when you tried to control your addiction, you begin to understand the power that addiction has had over your life. Acknowledging your powerlessness and recognizing the unmanageability in your life will help to prepare you to use the rest of the Twelve Steps.

Fill in the following chart for a clearer picture of your addiction. Either write your examples out in detail, or say a word or two that will remind you of the situation. Sharing your First Step with your group or your guides will allow them to help you in your recovery. Doing the worksheet and keeping it to yourself will not help your recovery. (See "Sharing Your First Step." If one aspect of addiction does not apply to you, just leave it blank.)

# Aspect of Addiction

Give three or more examples.

1. Obsessing or fantasizing about my addictive behavior

_____

_____

_____

_____

_____

_____

2. Trying to control my behavior

_____

_____

_____

_____

_____

_____

3. Lying, covering up, or minimizing my behavior

_____

_____

_____

_____

_____

_____

4. Trying to understand or rationalize my behavior

_____

_____

_____

_____

_____

_____

5. Effects on my physical health

_____

_____

_____

_____

_____

_____

6. Feeling guilty or shameful about my behaviors (or the other extreme—feeling defiant or prideful about my behaviors)

_____

_____

_____

_____

_____

_____

7. Effects on my emotional health

_____

_____

_____

_____

_____

_____

8. Effects on my social life

_____

_____

_____

_____

_____

9. Effects on my school or work life

_____

_____

_____

_____

_____

10. Effects on my character, morals, or values

_____

_____

_____

_____

_____

_____

11. Effects on my spirituality

_____

_____

_____

_____

_____

_____

12. Effects on my financial situation

_____

_____

_____

_____

_____

_____

13. Contact with the police or courts

14. Has my preoccupation led to insane or strange behavior?

15. Has my preoccupation led to loss of memory?

16. Has my preoccupation led to destructive behavior against self or others?

_____

_____

_____

_____

_____

_____

17. Has my preoccupation led to accidents or other dangerous situations?

_____

_____

_____

_____

_____

18. Do I keep overly or unnecessarily busy?

_____

_____

_____

_____

_____

_____

19. Do I feel depressed a lot of the time?

_____

_____

_____

_____

_____

_____

20. Am I able to share my feelings? If not, why not?

_____

_____

_____

_____

_____

_____

21. Have I changed my physical image to support my addiction?

_____

_____

_____

_____

_____

_____

22. Have I made promises to myself that I have broken?

_____

_____

_____

_____

_____

_____

23. Have I denied that I have a problem?

_____

_____

_____

_____

_____

24. Has my addiction affected my self-esteem?

_____

_____

_____

_____

_____

_____

25. Have I tried to relieve my pain about my behavior? How?

_____

_____

_____

_____

_____

_____

26. Have I tried to manipulate people into supporting my addiction? How?

_____

_____

_____

_____

_____

27. Have I given up my hobbies and interests? What were these?

_____

_____

_____

_____

# Powerlessness Inventory

List as many examples as you can think of that show how powerless you have been to stop your behavior. Remember, "powerless" means unable to stop the behavior despite obvious consequences. Be very explicit about types of behavior and frequencies. Start with your earliest example of being powerless, and conclude with your most recent. Generate at least thirty examples. By generating as many examples as possible, you will have added significantly to the depth of your understanding of your own powerlessness. Remember gentleness. You do not have to complete the list in one sitting. Add to the list as examples occur to you. When you finish this inventory, do not proceed until you have discussed it with one of your guides. The gentle way means you deserve support with each piece of significant work.

Example:  Sarah said she would leave in 1988 if I slipped again, and I did it anyway.

1. _____

_____

2. _____

_____

3. _____

_____

4. _____

_____

5. _____

_____

6. _____

_____

7. _____

_____

8. _____

_____

9. _____

_____

10. _____

_____

11. _____

_____

12. _____

_____

13. _____

_____

14. _____

_____

15. _____

_____

16. _____

_____

17. _____

_____

18. _____

_____

19. _____

_____

20. _____

_____

21. _____

_____

22. _____

_____

23. _____

_____

24. _____

_____

25. _____

_____

26. _____

_____

27. _____

_____

28. _____

_____

29. _____

_____

30. _____

_____

Those examples that happened most recently will make us feel our powerlessness the most. What are the most recent examples of powerlessness? Circle five that have happened recently.

# Unmanageability Inventory

List as many examples as you can think of that show how your life has become totally unmanageable because of your dependency. Remember, "unmanageability" means that your addiction created chaos and damage in your life. Again, when you finish this inventory, stop and talk to your guides. You deserve support.

Example: Got caught stealing in 1988 to support my addiction.

1. _____

2. _____

3. _____

4. _____

5. _____

6. _____

7. _____

8. _____

9. _____

10. _____

11. _____

12. _____

13. _____

14. _____

15. _____

16. _____

17. _____

18. _____

19. _____

20. _____

21. _____

22. _____

23. _____

24. _____

25. _____

26. _____

27. _____

28. _____

29. _____

30. _____

Those examples that happened most recently will make us feel our unmanageability the most. What are the most recent examples of unmanageability? Circle five that have happened for you in the last ten days. Circle five that have happened for you in the last thirty days.

# Step One for Coaddicts

> We admit we are powerless over coaddiction to
>
> _____
> (insert type of addiction)
> and that our lives have become unmanageable.

Acceptance of the First Step paves the way to recovery. When new to the Twelve Step program, most people find it easier to recognize the "sick" behavior of the addict than to recognize their own coaddictive behavior. As you grow to understand your own powerlessness and how unmanageable your life became when you tried to control the addiction, you begin to understand the power that addiction has had over your life. Acknowledging your powerlessness and recognizing your unmanageability will help prepare you to use the rest of the Twelve Steps.

Fill in the following chart for a clearer picture of your coaddiction. Either write your examples out in detail, or say a word or two that will remind you of the situation. Sharing your First Step with your group or your guides will allow them to help you in your recovery. If you have a hard time thinking of examples, ask them to help you. Doing the work-sheet and keeping it to yourself will not help your recovery. (See "Sharing Your First Step.") If any aspect of coaddiction does not apply to you, just leave it blank.

# Aspect of Coaddiction

Give three or more examples.

1.  Obsession about the addict's behavior

_____

_____

_____

_____

_____

2.  Ways I try to control the addict's behavior

_____

_____

_____

_____

_____

3.  Lying, covering up, or minimizing the addict's behavior

_____

_____

_____

_____

_____

4.  Attempts to figure out the addict's behavior

_____

_____

_____

_____

_____

5. Problems created by spending time with the addict when I should have focused on my own work, school, relationships, and so forth.

_____

_____

_____

_____

_____

6. Effects on my physical health

_____

_____

_____

_____

_____

7. Effects on my emotional health

_____

_____

_____

_____

_____

8. Effects on my social life

_____

_____

_____

_____

_____

9.   Effects on my school or work life

_____

_____

_____

_____

_____


10.  Gave in to the addict's ideas of character, morals, or values even
     when they were opposed to my own (effects on my character,
     morals, or values)

_____

_____

_____

_____

_____


11.  Effects on my spirituality

_____

_____

_____

_____

_____


12.  Effects on my financial situation

_____

_____

_____

_____

_____

13. Contact with the police or courts

_____

_____

_____

_____

_____

14. Has my preoccupation with the addict led to insane or strange behavior?

_____

_____

_____

_____

_____

15. Has my preoccupation with the addict led to loss of memory?

_____

_____

_____

_____

_____

16. Has my preoccupation with the addict led to destructive behavior against myself or others?

_____

_____

_____

_____

_____

17. Has my preoccupation with the addict led to accidents or other dangerous situations?

_____

_____

_____

_____

_____

18. Have I checked through the addict's mail, journals, or other personal effects?

_____

_____

_____

_____

19. Do I dress to accommodate the addict's wishes?

_____

_____

_____

_____

20. Do I lecture the addict for his or her problem?

_____

_____

_____

_____

21. Do I punish the addict? How?

_____

_____

_____

_____

_____

22. Do I blame myself for the addict's problem?

_____

_____

_____

_____

23. Do I use sex to get what I want?

_____

_____

_____

_____

24. Do I make excuses to not be sexual?

_____

_____

_____

_____

25. Do I attempt to persuade the addict to take care of himself or herself?

_____

_____

_____

_____

_____

26. Am I overly responsible or irresponsible?

_____

_____

_____

_____

27. Do I keep overly busy?

_____

_____

_____

_____

28. Do I feel depressed a lot of the time?

_____

_____

_____

_____

29. Am I able to deal with my feelings?

_____

_____

_____

_____

_____

30. Have I changed my physical image to please or displease the addict?

_____

_____

_____

_____

_____

31. Have I believed I could or should change the addict?

_____

_____

_____

_____

_____

32. Have I believed the addict's promises?

_____

_____

_____

_____

_____

33. Have I denied the addiction?

_____

_____

_____

_____

_____

34. Has the addiction affected my self-esteem?

_____

_____

_____

_____

_____

35. Do I try to relieve the addict's pain?

_____

_____

_____

_____

_____

36. Have I tried to manipulate the addict into changing?

_____

_____

_____

_____

_____

37. Have I given up my hobbies and interests?

_____

_____

_____

_____

_____

38. Has fear of rejection kept me in the relationship?

_____

_____

_____

_____

_____

39. Do I put the pieces back together after the addict creates chaos?

_____

_____

_____

_____

_____

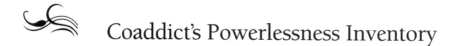 # Coaddict's Powerlessness Inventory

List as many examples as you can think of that show how powerless you have been to stop your behavior. Remember, "powerless" means unable to stop your behavior despite obvious negative consequences. Be very explicit about types of behavior and frequencies. Start with your earliest example of being powerless and conclude with your most recent. Generate at least thirty examples. By generating as many examples as possible, you will have added significantly to the depth of your understanding of your own powerlessness. Remember gentleness. You do not have to complete the list in one sitting. Add to the list as examples occur to you. When you finish this exercise, do not proceed until you have discussed it with one of your guides. The gentle way means you deserve support with each piece of work.

Example: I threatened to leave home in 1988 and he/she still did not stop drinking.

1. _____

_____

2. _____

_____

3. _____

_____

4. _____

_____

5. _____

_____

6. _____

_____

7. _____

   _____

8. _____

   _____

9. _____

   _____

10. _____

   _____

11. _____

   _____

12. _____

   _____

13. _____

   _____

14. _____

   _____

15. _____

   _____

16. _____

   _____

17. _____

   _____

18. _____

   _____

19. _____

   _____

20. _____

_____

21. _____

_____

22. _____

_____

23. _____

_____

24. _____

_____

25. _____

_____

26. _____

_____

27. _____

_____

28. _____

_____

29. _____

_____

30. _____

_____

Those examples that happened most recently will make you feel your powerlessness the most. What are the most recent examples of powerlessness? Circle five that have happened for you in the last ten days. Circle five that have happened for you in the last thirty days.

# Coaddict's Unmanageability Inventory

List as many examples as you can think of that show how your life has become totally unmanageable because of your codependency. Remember, "unmanageability" means that your coaddiction created chaos and damage in your life. Again, when you finish, stop and talk to your guides. You deserve support.

Example: In 1990, I had to get an extra job to support us because of his/her addiction.

1. _____

_____

2. _____

_____

3. _____

_____

4. _____

_____

5. _____

_____

6. _____

_____

7. _____

_____

8. _____

_____

9. _____

10. _____

11. _____

12. _____

13. _____

14. _____

15. _____

16. _____

17. _____

18. _____

19. _____

20. _____

21. _____

22. _____

_____

23. _____

_____

24. _____

_____

25. _____

_____

26. _____

_____

27. _____

_____

28. _____

_____

29. _____

_____

30. _____

_____

Those examples that happened most recently will make you feel your unmanageability the most. What are the most recent examples of unmanageability? Circle five that have happened for you in the last ten days. Circle five that have happened for you in the last thirty days.

# Sharing Your First Step

You have not fully taken your First Step unless you have shared it with others. One Twelve Step group has a tradition that, after ninety days in the program, a newcomer shares his or her first Step. The expectation helps remove procrastination. If you do a First Step in treatment, you may wish to do it again with your Twelve Step group. When you share your First Step, usually with a group, focus on telling about the depth and pain of your powerlessness, not necessarily your whole story. Choose incidents that are most moving to you. Get feedback and support from your guides about what to share. Remember, your goal is not to perform for others, but to help you see and accept your powerlessness. The more honest you are, the more relief you will feel.

The First Step invites you to share freely, holding little back. This is called "taking a Step" and means a fundamental acknowledgment of the illness and a surrender to a different life. Some people go through the motions of a First Step without actually taking the Step. They avoid the Step by sharing examples of their powerlessness and unmanageability, as if they are unrelated: They are detached from the impact of their illness. Taking the Step means clearly admitting the patterns of the illness and sharing the feelings that accompany the realization that you have been out of control. Healing occurs only when the Step goes past intellectual acceptance to emotional surrender.

Here's a comparison of some of the characteristics of *taking* versus *avoiding* a Step:

| Taking a Step | Avoiding a Step |
| --- | --- |
| Deliberate | Speedy |
| Thoughtful | Just reporting |
| Emotionally present | Emotionally absent |
| Feelings congruent with reality | Absence of feelings |
| Statements of ownership of feelings and responsibility for behavior | Blame, denial, projection |

| | |
|---|---|
| Events form patterns | Events seem isolated |
| Acceptance | Defensiveness |
| Acknowledge impact | Deny impact |
| Surrender to illness | Attempt to limit illness |
| See addiction as part of life | See addiction as something to be fixed |

---

Be aware of the tendency to become detached when telling your story. Try to remain open to both your own feelings and the group with whom you are sharing.

There are many reasons why people avoid, sometimes indefinitely, taking their First Step. Read the following items and see if any apply to you:

**Failure of courage**    To face an illness requires great courage. Some people are unable or unwilling to do it. If you find yourself thinking that you don't really need to do anything or that you can handle it by yourself, find someone in the program to support you in your fearful moments.

**Not witnessing a good First Step**    If you have never seen a First Step taken, then you have no real model of what to do. Watch someone else take the First Step, or ask your guide to talk to you about his or her First Step—how it was taken, what it meant.

**Inadequate preparation**    If you have not carefully prepared and consulted with your guides—that is, if you haven't carefully examined your own story—do not proceed. A First Step is not something you can do hastily.

**Denial of impact**    If you find yourself minimizing ("Things were not so bad") or wondering if you are making something out of nothing, it's time to go back over your story with your guides.

**Acting out**    Actively holding on to some aspect of the addiction or coaddiction, even in some very small way, will interfere with taking your First Step. Remember, you will not feel better until you completely stop your compulsive behavior.

**Holding on to a major secret**    Secrets most often involve shame, and shame will serve as a barrier to the self-acceptance necessary in taking a First Step. Share the secret with your guides or therapist before proceeding.

**Distrust of group**    Having confidence in your group is necessary in order for you to take the risks for your First Step work. If you do not feel comfortable in the group, talk to your guides about your options.

**Inadequate understanding of the Twelve Step program**    When you were brought into the program, someone explained how the Steps work. Each Step has a special purpose; all Twelve Steps taken in order will lead you to recovery. If you are still confused about the program, seek some help before attempting your Step work.

The concept of the "addictive personality shift" will help you here. Addicts and coaddicts acknowledge that in their illness, it seems like there are two people inside them—the real person who tries to live up to values and cares about people, and another person whose values and relationships are sacrificed to addictive obsession. This Jekyll-Hyde experience is very common. The addict within us all is, in the words of the "Big Book" of Alcoholics Anonymous, "cunning and baffling." Even being able to recognize the shift from when you are your true self and when your addict has taken over is an extremely helpful tool for detaching from your addict's power.

In terms of your First Step, your addict within will work hard to sabotage your efforts at an open sharing of your illness. List below five ways your addict might try to interfere with your First Step.

Example: Rationalization—"When I was drinking, my boss loved my work."

1.  _____

2.  _____

3.  _____

4.  _____

5.  _____

Sharing your Step work is crucial throughout the program.

# Guide Reactions

This page is reserved for comments from your guides about your progress on your First Step. It is a place where they can write their encouragement, support, and reactions. This, too, is part of your history. Completing this page and the other guide reaction pages in this workbook is optional, not a requirement. Remember, though, that part of recovery is learning to accept support and praise, and this is a good time to begin.

Guides write here:

_____

_____

_____

_____

_____

_____

_____

_____

_____

_____

_____

_____

_____

Guide name: _____

Date: _____

# The Serenity Prayer

No better statement of our need to reestablish balance in our lives can be found than in the Serenity Prayer.

## God grant me the serenity . . .

Serenity means that I no longer recoil from the past, live in jeopardy because of my present behavior, or worry about the unknown future. I seek regular times to re-create myself and I avoid those times of depletion that make me vulnerable to despair and to old self-destructive patterns.

## to accept the things I cannot change . . .

Accepting change means that I do not cause suffering for myself by clinging to that which no longer exists. All that I can count on is that nothing will be stable—except how I respond to the transforming cycles in my life of birth, growth, and death.

## the courage to change the things I can . . .

Giving up my attempts to control outcomes does not require that I give up my boundaries or my best efforts. It does mean my most honest appraisal of the limits of what I can do.

## and the wisdom to know the difference.

Wisdom becomes the never forgotten recognition of all those times when it seemed there was no way out, and new paths opened up like miracles in my life.

# Reflections
## on the
## First Step

On this page, and on pages like it at the end of each chapter, you are asked to stop and summarize your feelings about the Step you have just taken. It's important for you to appreciate the ground you have already covered, as well as to consider ways to keep from losing that ground.

Now that you have taken and shared your First Step, reflect on what it means to you. Reflect also on the Serenity Prayer. What things can you do to make the philosophy contained in this prayer part of your daily life?

# Celebrating Your Progress

Congratulations on completing your First Step, so crucial to your recovery. If this Step has left you open to shame attacks, you may want to spend a lot of time with people in the program who will help you stay on the gentle path. *Suggestion:* Create a celebration for yourself to mark your progress!

What are some of the gentle, healthy ways you can celebrate the new beginning you have made? What are some of the ways you can celebrate your progress as you work the program during the coming weeks and months?

# Step Two

Came to believe that a Power greater than ourselves could restore us to sanity.

# Step Three

Made a decision to turn our will and our lives over to the care of God *as we understood Him*.

I was raised Catholic. It was Christmas time, and I was in the first grade. The priest of our little country parish called my mother and asked if I could serve as an altar boy on Christmas morning. I expressed some fear, because I had never done it before, nor had I been through the "altar boy training program." He told me to come early that morning and he would show me all I needed to know.

On that fateful morning I dutifully showed up early. My mother, thrilled at the prospect of my serving at Mass on Christmas morning, had invited her five sisters and their families to join us. This had now become a high-drama event. My fear was escalating. Old Father Yanny, however, was very reassuring. There were only two things I had to remember. One was when I was to move the "Book" from one side of the altar to the other. The second was to ring a set of bells whenever he put his right hand on the altar. In those days, the bell was a signal to the congregation to kneel, sit, or stand at different points in the liturgy.

Father Yanny was getting on in years. He probably wasn't aware that he often leaned on the altar to steady himself—using his right hand. When he leaned, I rang. When I rang, the congregation moved. I had that church going up and down, up and down. My mother was mortified. My aunts thought it was great, and they tell the story to this day.

Whether it was "right" or not, the people moved when the bell rang. As an adult, I think of that experience as a metaphor about religion. For many, it often seems like a forced or meaningless motion. How many of us have become detached from a spiritual life because the ritual does not fit our lives?

I remember a patient who told this story about family week. It was Sunday morning and his spouse was attending service in the church across the road. He sat in his room, looking at that church, knowing she was inside. He was moved by her faithfulness, especially about how important their relationship was to her. With that emotion he had a flash of insight about how he had put "faith" in the wrong things as part of his illness. With the tears that came, he felt connected to his partner and the presence of his Higher Power. For most, the story is the same. Spiritual things happen when you admit suffering.

Ultimately, this question of meaning is a spiritual one. Steps Two and Three ask, Whom do you trust? Whom or what do you have faith in? How much you trust others often parallels your trust in a Higher Power. If you have trouble accepting help from others and insist on handling things alone, chances are you will resist the help of a Higher Power in your life. Many addicts who have worked the program realize that if they refuse help after admitting that they are powerless and damaged, they will remain stuck in their insanity.

The First Step asks you to admit that you have an illness. Steps Two and Three ask you to confront the question of what gives your life meaning. Without meaning in your life, your addiction and coaddiction can grow and thrive. Without meaning, you cannot establish the priorities that help you restore the balance, focus, and self-responsibility you seek.

Six things will make these Steps easier:

1. **Spiritual Care Inventory**—Helps you identify obstacles to completing Step Two and Step Three.

2. **Loss of Reality Inventory**—Helps you focus on your priorities.

3. **Paths to Spirituality**—There are many ways to experience spirituality. This exercise allows you to reflect on some spiritual moments you may have experienced but hadn't identified as spiritual.

4. **Spiritual Path Affirmations**—These affirmations will help replace the negative messages and ideas we learned about God with positive ones.

5. **One-Year-to-Live Fantasy**—An exercise in confronting your own death. Provides perspective on the spirituality and meaningfulness of your life.

6. **Letter to Your Higher Power**—Gives you a concrete way to express your spiritual decisions.

Remember to include your guides in this process.

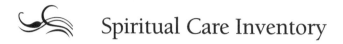 # Spiritual Care Inventory

## Openness to Spirituality—A Self-Assessment

Consider the following:

In a grocery store, when searching for something you cannot find, do you (check one):

❑ Keep searching until you find it.

❑ Ask for help.


When putting something together from a kit, do you (check one):

❑ Follow directions carefully.

❑ Quickly go through the instructions only when you get stuck.

❑ Figure it out for yourself.


When you are personally in pain and need support, do you usually:

❑ Talk to people immediately.

❑ Wait until the crisis is over and then tell people.

❑ Get through it the best way you can without help.


As you responded to these situations, did you discover a pattern of not letting yourself be helped? Often addicts and coaddicts rely solely on themselves.

As an addict or coaddict, you have relied on your obsessions to deal with pain and difficulty. You may have learned not to depend on people for help, care, and support. It is probable that you learned not to accept help based on the way your primary caregivers treated you as a child. Consider the following list of people. How did they affect your ability to receive help? Did they support you when you made a mistake? Did they show you how to do things, or did they expect you to know without being taught?

Your father

_____

_____

_____

_____

_____

_____

Your mother

_____

_____

_____

_____

_____

Brothers and sisters

_____

_____

_____

_____

_____

_____

Other significant adults (specify)

_____

_____

_____

_____

_____

Teacher (specify)

_____

_____

_____

_____

_____

Employers (specify)

_____

_____

_____

_____

_____

Clergy (specify)

_____

_____

_____

_____

Describe your feelings when it becomes necessary for you to ask for help:

| | | | |
|---|---|---|---|
| beginning | scared | uncertain | tentative |
| learner | vulnerable | rebellious | challenging |
| resisting | nontrusting | questioning | testing |
| loner | unique | free | separate |
| individualist | detached | cooperative | nurturing |
| guiding | assisting | directing | reliable |

From the list of twenty-four words above, select the six words that most aptly describe you. Now these same twenty-four words are arranged below in terms of dependence, counterdependence, independence, and interdependence. Find the six words you selected above and circle them again. Have you circled three or more words in any one category?

| Dependence | Counterdependence | Independence | Interdependence |
|---|---|---|---|
| beginning | rebellious | loner | cooperative |
| scared | challenging | unique | nurturing |
| uncertain | resisting | free | guiding |
| tentative | nontrusting | separate | assisting |
| learner | questioning | individualist | directing |
| vulnerable | testing | detached | reliable |

The terms can be defined as follows:

**Dependence**—We need and want help.

**Counterdependence**—We need help but resist it.

**Independence**—We are self-sufficient and do not need help.

**Interdependence**—We give and get help to and from others.

# Higher Power Attitude Index

Now that you know how you normally react when you need help from others, you may take a spiritual attitude inventory. Accepting your reality does not mean making excuses for continuing with your insanity. It means you recognize where you are and how you need to change to become responsible for yourself.

Circle the six words that best describe how you understand God or your Higher Power:

| | | | |
|---|---|---|---|
| judgmental | strict | negative | rigid |
| cruel | arbitrary | caring | trustable |
| loving | purposeful | compassionate | predictable |
| distant | indifferent | uncaring | nonattentive |
| absent | disengaged | hoax | unreal |
| nonexistent | fanciful | imaginary | joke |

Your perceptions of a Higher Power have evolved over the years. Before you can be truly reflective about a Higher Power, you need to clarify your attitudes toward God. Four ways of viewing God exist for many of us:

**A punishing God** who punishes our mistakes but does not reward or help.

**An accepting God** who accepts that we fail and cares anyway.

**A noninvolved God** who is detached and unconcerned with our lives.

**A nonexistent God** from whom no help is available.

From the list of twenty-four words, you selected six words that most aptly described your perceptions of God. These twenty-four words are arranged into four columns, each representing a different view of God: punishing, accepting, noninvolved, or nonexistent. Circle the six words you selected previously. Does any category include three or more words?

| Punishing | Accepting | Noninvolved | Nonexistent |
|-----------|-----------|-------------|-------------|
| judgmental | caring | distant | hoax |
| strict | trustable | indifferent | unreal |
| negative | loving | uncaring | nonexistent |
| rigid | purposeful | nonattentive | fanciful |
| cruel | compassionate | absent | imaginary |
| arbitrary | predictable | disengaged | joke |

Are there patterns in the words you selected?

_____

_____

_____

_____

_____

Are there any correlations between the adjectives that describe your Higher Power and the descriptions of how the caregivers in your life helped you?

_____

_____

_____

_____

_____

_____

How have your perceptions of God or your Higher Power changed over time?

_____

_____

_____

_____

_____

_____

_____

_____

How does your current mode of accepting help (dependent, counterdependent, independent, and interdependent) fit with your perception of God or your Higher Power?

_____

_____

_____

_____

_____

_____

_____

_____

Name the five persons who most influenced your attitudes toward God or your Higher Power:

1. _____

2. _____

3. _____

4. _____

5. _____

Do they have anything in common?

_____

_____

_____

_____

_____

_____

What obstacles does your religious background or upbringing give you for trusting a Higher Power?

_____

_____

_____

_____

_____

_____

What strengths does your religious background or upbringing give you for trusting in a Higher Power?

_____

_____

_____

_____

_____

_____

_____

Based on what you have learned about recovery so far, how do you see the "turning over" process of Step Three? What are the things that might prevent you, emotionally and intellectually, from accepting the help of a Higher Power?

_____

_____

_____

_____

_____

_____

_____

_____

_____

_____

_____

_____

_____

_____

_____

_____

_____

_____

_____

_____

In what ways do you see a Higher Power working in your life now?

1. _____

   _____

2. _____

   _____

3. _____

   _____

4. _____

   _____

5. _____

   _____

6. _____

   _____

7. _____

   _____

8. _____

   _____

9. _____

   _____

10. _____

    _____

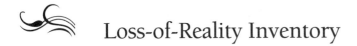 # Loss-of-Reality Inventory

Even after recognizing the unmanageability of our lives in the First Step, many of us still do not want to use the word *insanity* to describe our own behavior and thinking. Denial and delusion come from addictive and coaddictive, impaired thinking. Considering that insanity involves some loss of touch with reality, addicts and coaddicts need to regain perspective on what is real and what is not. Spirituality will continue to elude us if we persist in delusion. The following are three descriptive categories of reality loss.

1.  **No reality** You "lose" your memory from a combination of factors, including obsession, overextension, exhaustion, or anxiety and intoxication. Or, you lose contact with here-and-now events because of the same combination. One recovering coaddict described her experience with loss of reality: "We were newlyweds in our first year of marriage. One night my husband was arrested for voyeurism. I functioned perfectly through that embarrassing night, and when I awoke the next day I had forgotten all about it. And I continued to have no memory of it for thirty years, until two years ago, when I started my own recovery. Now I can remember every detail, the colors, what I wore, every minute."

    Reflect on your own experience with no reality and loss of memories:

    _____

    _____

    _____

    _____

    _____

    _____

2.  **Distortion of reality** Reality is blurred because of the power the addiction has over you. Think of things you thought were true because your addict wanted them to be true. Or, think of how you have distorted reality because of faulty beliefs. (If you start with a faulty belief, such as "Women have to be seduced in order to enjoy sex," your thought processes will naturally be faulty as well. You may believe, for example, that seduction is the only way to get sexual needs met.)

Reflect on your own distortions of reality:

_____

_____

_____

_____

_____

_____

_____

_____

_____

_____

A group in Colorado developed a distorted core belief exercise called "I'm only lovable if...." Examples are "I'm only lovable if I'm sexual," "I'm only lovable if I'm perfect," "I'm only lovable if I don't ask for anything."

Complete your own "I'm only lovable if..." delusion exercise:

I'm only lovable if _____

_____

I'm only lovable if _____

_____

I'm only lovable if _____

_____

I'm only lovable if _____

_____

3.   **Ignoring reality**   When you ignore reality, you fail to assess risks accurately. Or you overcome the recognition that recent experiences were disastrous by your compulsion to repeat them. An addict knows the penalties but goes ahead and does the act anyway. Risking unsafe sex, financial overextension, job loss, arrest, car accidents, loss of marriage, and legal consequences are all examples.

Describe specific examples when you ignored reality and suffered consequences:

_____

_____

_____

_____

_____

_____

_____

_____

_____

_____

Describe specific examples when you ignored reality and escaped the consequences:

_____

_____

_____

_____

_____

_____

_____

Now reflect on your losses of reality. When you needed help, whom did you ask? When you asked your Higher Power or other people for help, was your request based on reality?

_____

_____

_____

_____

_____

_____

_____

_____

_____

_____

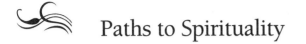 Paths to Spirituality

Across world religions and throughout the history of human experience with the Divine, we find certain universally recognized strategies to nurturing spirituality. While each person's experience is unique, these ways of approaching life maximize our availability to spiritual presence. Each of the following is a common path others have taken. We suggest you use each thought as a meditation to reflect on and journal about over the next ten days.

1. **Be as a child.** The master said, "Unless you are as one of these children," you will miss the path. The goal here is not to be naive, but to be open. Children live fully in the moment. Adults are distracted by the past and concerned about the future; children live in the now. Adults focus on what is practical; children focus on what is. Every parent has had a chance to see through a child's eyes and marvel at the world adults often miss. Children are totally engaged in what is happening around them. They want to explore and understand everything, immediately, with all their senses. It is easy to be intimate with children because they are so vulnerable and open. Spirituality is about intimacy—closeness and appreciation of oneself, others, and a Higher Power.

For some of us, to be vulnerable and open was to risk exploitation. So we built defenses and coping mechanisms that split us off from our experiences. It is partly how we lost our spiritual connection. In the safety of recovery, the challenge is to reclaim our vulnerability and openness so we can be present to the world.

Reflect on what you would have to do to be more "present" in your life. Record your thoughts here:

**2. Connect with the earth.** The senses are the gateway to a spiritual life. They put us in touch with the complexity, beauty, and wonder of creation. Reflect on the most peaceful and serene moments of your life. Notice that nature was somehow usually involved. Mountains, seas, sunsets, and woods create awe and tranquillity. It is this peace which connects us to the larger picture of the universe.

Native peoples are sustained spiritually by connection with the planet. They live with the immediacy of growing things. What they eat, they hunt or gather. They have a sense of what had to die that they might live. So they respect creation but are matter-of-fact about life and death. They do not miss the central reality of their existence. They are part of a larger ecology with intelligence and purpose. To survive means to acknowledge the larger rhythms of the planet.

Contemporary peoples tend to be removed from these life realities. They create buildings for spiritual life because they experience only the community, not the connection with nature. They often are not aware of where their food comes from, nor do they have any sense of its life—or where they fit in the food chain. They fear death and see nature as something to be overcome. Then they agonize over their existential aloneness.

For many recovering people, the beginning of a spiritual life started with some reconnection with the planet. What ways are available to you? Record them here. Pick one to do today, and others to do in the next weeks:

**3. Develop a beginner's mind.** When a Zen warrior or monk practices "emptying the mind," it literally means discarding preoccupations and fears and being in the moment. This means emptying the mind of all preconceived, conditioned thought or prejudice—to be totally open to the moment and what it may teach. The beginner learns to appreciate the moment for what it is—a new experience. To be most responsive—whether for battle or discernment—one gives no thought to the outcomes.

Joseph Campbell and others who have studied the hero's myths in many lands notice that a similar process is central in every hero's journey. The hero comes to a point where he or she must stop worrying about what to do or how to overcome the obstacles in the way, and just do what needs to be done. Right action comes by taking the next step. But first the hero must surrender or submit to the teaching of a spiritual guide or mentor. Through this process, the hero learns the inner discernment necessary to make wise decisions. The relationship between Luke Skywalker and Yoda clearly reflects this process. Not until Luke fully sets aside his pride and surrenders does he experience the full power of The Force.

Initiation rites in primitive cultures mark an individual's passage from one state of being to a higher level. The initiate (or beginner) never knows exactly what is going to happen, but allows designated members of the community to direct the ritual process. Usually this surrender involves pain, just as it does for the hero. The initiate's suffering taps into new strengths, and new destinies emerge. The initiate is fundamentally changed.

Sadly, we lack these rites in contemporary culture. Recovering people, however, have much in common with the initiate, the hero, and the Zen Master. Steps One through Three demand surrender without knowing what will happen. With surrender comes pain and transformation. Recovery is like the hero's journey or the initiate's ordeal. Once we have begun, there is no going back. With each turn in the road, we must empty our minds once again. If we are to fully experience the unfolding reality of our lives, there is no other path.

List here the obstacles in your life to the "beginner's" mind:

_____

_____

_____

_____

_____

_____

_____

_____

_____

_____

**4. Access your own wisdom.** Emptying ourselves of distractions, preoccupations, and obsessions allows us to connect with who we really are. Henri Nouwen, the famous theologian, described this early stage of spiritual life as the "conversion of loneliness into solitude." It means discovering what Dietrich Bonhoeffer called, "the ground of our being." It is finding the sacred within us. When we are true to ourselves, we are most spiritual. That means tuning in to our own authentic voice.

How do we do that? Think of your own life experience. Think of the times you had an intuition that something was not going to work out, but you did it anyway. And when that turned out to be a disaster, you said, "If only I had listened to myself." Carl Jung talked about a larger consciousness that we can tap into with our intuition—if we would listen. This is called "discernment"—the ability to see clearly what is, especially in those situations when we have no rules, laws, or prior experience to direct us. This is where divine guidance and trusting ourselves meet. All heroes come to this crossroads where they do not know the outcome but must act.

To cultivate discernment, keep a regular journal, develop a daily mediation routine, listen to music that makes you feel like yourself, and read what helps your insight and sense of self. There is no magic about this process. If you work at it, your true voice—the one that is in harmony with the larger universe—will become clear.

List five times you have ignored your inner voice:

1. _____

2. _____

3. _____

4. _____

5. _____

In what ways can you deepen your own discernment?

1. _____

2. _____

3. _____

4. _____

5. _____

**5. Care for your body.** Loving and nurturing your body is a metaphor for every spiritual task you face and is the primary spiritual act. Jigaro Kano, the revered founder of modern judo, thought that physical discipline was a gateway to spiritual growth. Mastering the technique was the least important part. Facing your fear, emptying yourself, trusting your own voice, letting go of control, having faith in outcomes, connecting with a larger purpose, deriving meaning from the struggle— that is the primary work of the athlete. Kano also taught that physical development was a lifetime commitment—not a casual task, nor only for the young. Like the Greeks, he saw physical exercise as an essentially spiritual discipline that we must practice until we die. In the West, we tend to see fitness as an optional health concern that can be a low priority in a busy schedule. We make physical fitness into a competition and confer status symbols—Olympic gold medals or multi-million-dollar baseball contracts—on a few gifted athletes. Occasionally, when someone refers to the runner's high or the "Zen" of weightlifting, we glimpse the more profound connection between mind and body. When we separate these positive experiences from the rest of life, we split the two and add to our spiritual damage.

Here is the reality: Our body is the primary vehicle through which we experience our world. As the custodian of the organism in which we reside, we must nurture and tend to it. We must stretch and grow. Anything less splits us off from one of the central sources of awe about creation: our bodies. It is the most concrete way we have to embrace the spiritual struggle that teaches us. A contemplative life is not an inactive one. It requires the gentle but continuous flow of our energy.

List obstacles to an active physical life:

1. _____

2. _____

3. _____

4. _____

5. _____

6. _____

7. _____

8. _____

9. _____

10. _____

_____

How many of these obstacles could be restated as obstacles to a spiritual life? (Example: not enough time.) Put a check after each one that would be true of both. Record your reflection about the commonalities:

_____

_____

_____

_____

_____

_____

_____

**6. Search for the circles.** The circle is a sacred symbol of connectedness. Plants, animals, and people decay and die and are replaced by new growth and the miracle of birth. Seasons recycle the earth. Everything and everyone is nestled in this larger connectedness. In central Africa, the symbol is a sacred snake configured so it consumes its own tail. Native American peoples used the sacred hoop to signify the four points of the compass. Christians have used the circle to describe life, death, and resurrection.

Theologian Paul Tillich described sin and grace from this perspective. He said that sin was about action that separated you from yourself, others, and God. Grace originated in connection with yourself, others, and God. The Navajo use the phrase "being in harmony." When we truly experience this source of belonging and connecting, we find extraordinary meaning in our lives. We can understand the words of Chief Seattle when he said, "You must teach your children that the ground beneath their feet is the ashes of their grandfathers."

Holding hands in a Twelve Step meeting and saying the Serenity Prayer is the first experience of reconnection for many recovering people. In time they grow to realize that at any time, night or day, there is a group somewhere saying that prayer. With further understanding, they realize that each person's struggle is important to all the other members of the group, and ultimately, to all the groups. The recovery process itself is a rebirth out of the ashes. And with each person who makes it, the whole is better. In fact, the entire planet is better.

On the next page, draw a picture of your support community, using circles. Do not use any words, just indicate connections. After completing the drawing, what do you notice?

**7. Find spiritual guides.** In our obsessions, we are fiercely committed to handling things on our own. If we consult others, the temptation is to give them only part of the story or share after the crisis is over. To allow someone to see the full extent of our despair when it is happening in all of its untidy, ugly, and searing reality is a tremendous leap of faith. We resist it, since to acknowledge the wound is to experience the pain. We are not expected to do this alone. Absolutely essential to a spiritual path is allowing ourselves the gift of help.

Spiritual guides come mainly in three ways. First, we find trusted persons who can teach us from their own wounding experiences. We tell them how it is for us. Their perspective and support ease the pain. They give us concrete ways to connect with our Higher Power. Sponsors, clergy, therapists, mentors, teachers, elders—all come in this category.

Second, we seek spiritual community. We find spiritual guidance in groups of people—Twelve Step fellowships, religious communities, men's and women's groups—also committed to walking a spiritual path. We will connect with spiritual guides wherever we find that we are not alone, and there are celebrations and symbols of our progress together.

Finally, we are open to guidance from others around us every day. The answers to our struggles are surrounding us if we listen to the possibilities. An offhand comment by someone may have been exactly what we needed to hear. Watching some creature live its life can be a metaphor for what we need—if we allow for the possibility. Asking questions like *How am I like the wolf, the turtle or the wren?* or *How does an animal greet pain, make herself comfortable, or use caution?* opens us to a deeper connection with the natural world—and ourselves. By analogy, we can meditate on the significance for our own lives.

Reflect for a moment on how you receive direction in your life. Do you seek it, using it as a way to expand your potential? Or do you resist it and see it as an intrusion? Who have been your guides so far? How well have you used them? Record your thoughts below:

_____

_____

_____

_____

_____

_____

**8. Accept pain as a teacher.** All of us have suffered. For some, it is caused by the trauma of betrayal, neglect, or exploitation. Sometimes the source is a cataclysm that seems to have no purpose beyond destruction. All of us experience change. So we have the grief of that which is no more. A Buddhist definition of suffering is "clinging to that which changes." Twelve Step programs basically teach us to adopt an existential view of change and suffering. It is best summarized in the Serenity Prayer:

*"God grant me the serenity*
*to accept the things I cannot change,*
*the courage to change the things I can,*
*and the wisdom to know the difference."*

Viktor Frankl, in his study of survivors of the Nazi concentration camps, noticed that those who survived had a common quality: the ability to transform suffering into meaning. Spirituality is about meaning and asking questions like *Why do bad things happen?* and *Who is in charge of it all?* We tend to war against difficult issues when they surface in our lives. We talk of "my fight against cancer." Part of a spiritual path involves learning to "see my illness as a teacher."

Suffering simply is. It's not fair, right, or wrong. It simply is. However, how I respond is critical. How I take action, how I grow, and how I become a more spiritual person is the most important thing. Remember the fundamental lesson the Greeks taught in their tragedies. The hero typically suffered from a tragic flaw—hubris, or the sin of pride. Oedipus and the other great heroes refused to accept their human limitations and made themselves into gods. Whenever they ignored their own limitations and wounds, however, they met a tragic fate. Our wounds help us to accept our humanness and be open to the lessons provided for us.

Make a list of five painful experiences in your life. Then list some reasons why you have come to value those experiences.

1. _____

2. _____

3. _____

4. _____

5. _____

Think of your struggles. What are the lessons for you now? Record your thoughts here:

**9. Develop spiritual habits.** Recovering people can often remember traumatic experiences in childhood that altered their lives. But it was the daily experience of living in the family which had the greatest impact. So it happens with spiritual life. Spiritual experiences occur that alter one's life. But it is the daily spiritual practices that bring spiritual depth. St. Paul told us of his "conversion" experience on the road to Damascus. Yet it is he who cautions that "every day we are surrendered unto death." Native Americans echo this belief when they say that the only thing one needs to do each day is pray.

Another way to view daily spirituality is to think of it as a relationship. Relationships are not sustained by dramatic encounters, but by daily efforts which over time deepen the relationship. To develop a spiritual relationship with your Higher Power takes commitment and time. Having a regular routine makes a dramatic difference. Starting is hard. We do not see results immediately. Sponsors often suggest that we "act as if." Allow the time. Start with simple readings and meditations. Diets, exercise programs, developing new skills—all those things are hard at first. But regular, daily work makes a difference.

One of the key discoveries is that you can make your own rituals and prayers. While many participate in spiritual communities, each person's journey is unique. So we can add our own symbols, our own patterns of meditation. We discover reflections that help us and modify them for our own use. Spirituality evolves from groping when we are in trouble to a daily extension of our internal life.

Write below your daily "spiritual recipe." Describe it as if you were explaining it to someone who wanted to practice what you do. If you are not doing anything currently, describe what "recipe" might work for you.

**10. Work on Steps.** Each of the Twelve Steps contributes to our spiritual life. Here is how:

**Step One** confronts the paradox of our addictive and coaddictive processes. We feel powerful when, in fact, we are powerless and need help.

**Step Two** challenges our grandiosity and reminds us that we are limited human beings.

**Step Three** underlines our efforts to control when we need to take responsibility only for ourselves and leave the rest to our Higher Power.

**Step Four** takes the energy out of the shame that separates us from ourselves, others, and our Higher Power. It brings acceptance.

**Step Five** asks us to break through the paralyzing fear that prevents us from receiving forgiveness and faith.

**Step Six** attacks our perfectionism, allowing us to experience our wounds so that we might heal.

**Step Seven** asks us to give up our willfulness so that we might allow change to work in our lives and to begin grieving.

**Step Eight** asks us to exchange our pride for honesty.

**Step Nine** challenges us to stop seeking approval and to pursue integrity by making amends for harm we have caused.

**Step Ten** makes a daily prescription to set aside our defenses and admit our errors.

**Step Eleven** asks us to trade the magical thinking of escapism for the realities of a spiritual life even though they are difficult.

**Step Twelve** tells us to trade in our martyrlike victim roles and share the changes in our lives with others with similar problems.

The following chart summarizes the effect of the Steps upon addictive or coaddictive behavior:

| In our addiction we were | | In our recovery we seek |
|---|---|---|
| Deluded | Step One | Reality |
| Grandiose | Step Two | A sense of limitations |
| Controlling | Step Three | Faith in others |
| Shameful | Step Four | Self-worth |
| Fearful | Step Five | Forgiveness |
| Perfectionism | Step Six | Healing of brokenness |
| Willful | Step Seven | Letting go |
| Prideful | Step Eight | Honesty |
| Approval seeking | Step Nine | Integrity |
| Defensive | Step Ten | Responsibility |
| Escapist | Step Eleven | Connectedness |
| Self-suffering | Step Twelve | Witnessing our path |

The "Big Book" of Alcoholics Anonymous tells us that if we do these things, certain "promises" will be fulfilled:

> We are going to know a new freedom and a new happiness. We will not regret the past nor wish to shut the door on it. We will comprehend the word *serenity*, and we will know peace. No matter how far down the scale we have gone, we will see how our experience can benefit others. That feeling of uselessness and self-pity will disappear. We will lose interest in selfish things and gain interest in our fellows. Self-seeking will slip away. Our whole attitude and outlook upon life will change. Fear of people and of economic insecurity will leave us. We will intuitively know how to handle situations that used to baffle us. We will suddenly realize that God is doing for us what we could not do for ourselves.

What reactions or reflections do you have about the "promises" for yourself? If you were to write your own version of the "promises" to pass on to others, what would you write? Record them here:

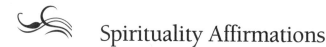

# Spirituality Affirmations

The following list of suggested affirmations will help you reprogram yourself for spiritual openness. Read them each day, or tape record these positive messages and listen to them before falling asleep at night. Select from the list the affirmations that have meaning for you, and add some of your own. Gradually, as you repeat these affirmations to yourself, you will begin to experience and internalize your inner truth. Affirmations are a spiritual gift you can give to yourself.

*Each moment of my day is filled with openness and vulnerability to the world around me.*

*I am connected to my planet. I experience the sky, the wind, the rain, and all the elements of my environment. I am aware of the cycle of life. Each day brings greater awareness of my place in this universe.*

*With an empty mind, I take in each moment as a new experience. Each moment in recovery brings transformation.*

*I have an inner, true voice that is in harmony with the universe. Each day I develop greater acuity and discernment in interpreting my voice's clear messages to me.*

*My body is my primary vehicle for embracing the awe of my world. Each day I nurture and tend to it. Stretching my body brings energy, strength, and confidence to face my struggles.*

*I am connected to the past, present, and future. What has gone before me is part of me and I will be a part of what goes on after me. I am part of the circle of my community. As we are all connected to the past, present, and future, we are all connected to each other.*

*I am open to the spiritual guidance of others. My spiritual guides are those I love and trust, those I respect, those who have a message for me and those who offer symbols to help me on my journey.*

*My wounds are my teachers. I am open to their lessons.*

*I practice my spirituality daily. My spirituality is a daily extension of my internal life.*

## I Affirm the Promises for Myself

*I know a new freedom and happiness.*

*I embrace my past.*

*I comprehend the word serenity and know peace.*

*I can see how my experience can benefit others.*

*That feeling of uselessness and self-pity has disappeared.*

*As I lose interest in selfish things, I gain interest in my fellows.*

*Self-seeking has slipped away.*

*My whole attitude and outlook upon life is changing.*

*Fear of people and economic insecurity has left.*

*I intuitively know how to handle situations that used to baffle me.*

*I realize that God is doing for me what I could not do for myself.*

Create affirmations that are meaningful to you:

_____

_____

_____

_____

_____

# One-Year-to-Live Fantasy

Reclaiming reality starts with a clear sense of our limitations as human beings. But we live in a culture that denies these limitations. We are constantly invited to overextend ourselves—for example, to spend more than we earn, work more than we need to, or eat more than we should. We live as if there were no end. We literally deny our own mortality.

A powerful exercise that can show you your own limitations is to picture your own death. Looking at death provides vital perspectives about what gives your life meaning, what priorities you are ignoring, and who your Higher Power is.

Record the following fantasy on a tape recorder, then set aside some uninterrupted time to listen to it and answer the questions provided at the end. Pause for ten to fifteen seconds where indicated before you continue. Make sure you are physically comfortable. If you do not have a tape recorder, you may read the fantasy, or have your guide or a close friend read it to you.

## Fantasy

*Imagine that you are in your physician's office. What does it look, smell, and feel like? Your doctor comes in and tells you that results from the tests are in. You have a terminal illness. All the other doctors consulted agree. They think you will maintain your physical ability for about a year—but at the end of the year you will die. [pause]*

*Imagine your first reactions as you walk out of the office. What do you do? [pause] How do you spend those first few hours and days? [pause] Do you tell anyone? [pause]*

*As you start to adjust to your dying, do you change your life? Stop work? Do something different? [pause]*

*Maybe you want to do something different. Perhaps you wish to travel. Where would you go? Picture yourself traveling. Whom would you bring with you? [pause]*

*Perhaps you might want to do things you have never done before. Activities like skydiving, scuba diving, race car driving seemed too dangerous before, but now it doesn't make any difference. What have you always wanted to do but been afraid to do? [pause] Picture yourself doing this. Who is with you? [pause]*

*Almost all of us have "unfinished" parts of our lives: a book we are writing, a family room to finish, a family project like getting the family album in order for the kids. What unfinished projects would be important enough to finish before you die? [pause] Imagine yourself doing them. [pause]*

*For some of us, the unfinished parts include things not said to others—like "I'm sorry" or "I love you." Picture yourself saying the things you would need to say before you die. [pause]*

*It's now about three months before you die. You can start to feel your health fail. While you can still function, you decide to try one last thing. What would that be? [pause] What would be one of the last things you would want to do before you die? [pause] Who is with you? [pause]*

*It's now a matter of weeks before you die. Where do you go to die? [pause] Your home? A family farm? A lake? The mountains? The city? [pause] How do you spend those last days? [pause] Who is with you? [pause]*

*As you think over the events of this last year of your life, what were the most significant ones for you? [pause] In fact, think of these and all the events of your life. Which stand out now as the things that made life worthwhile? [pause]*

*As you reflect on these events, be aware that you are working on this workbook. And you are very much alive. Be aware of your current surroundings. Wiggle your fingers and toes to bring yourself all the way back to the present, and become ready to move on to your next activity.*

## About the Fantasy . . .

Often this fantasy helps people touch their own grief about losses in their lives. If you feel sad, do not avoid the feelings. Rather, use them and let them support you in coming to terms with your losses. Sharing the fantasy and your feelings with your guides can deepen your understanding of the issues the fantasy raises. First, record the details of your fantasy in the space provided. Then answer the questions that follow.

Your first reactions:

_____

_____

_____

_____

_____

_____

Changes you would make in your life:

_____

_____

_____

_____

_____

_____

_____

New things you would try:

_____

_____

_____

_____

_____

Unfinished things you want to complete:

_____

_____

_____

_____

_____

Things you need to say before you die:

_____

_____

_____

_____

_____

Describe your last fling:

_____

_____

_____

_____

_____

_____

Spiritual preparations:

_____

_____

_____

_____

_____

_____

Where and how you would spend your last days:

_____

_____

_____

_____

_____

_____

Throughout the fantasy there were key moments involving significant persons in your life. Whom did you involve and what did you learn about your relationship priorities?

_____

_____

_____

_____

_____

_____

During the fantasy, you may have found yourself doing things significantly differently from how you live now. Why would this be so? If they were so important to get done, what prevents you from doing them now?

_____

_____

_____

_____

_____

_____

How do you feel about facing your own death?

_____

_____

_____

_____

_____

_____

Thinking about death provides a way to look at what is real and what is important in our lives. How have your ideas of what is important and real to you changed after experiencing this death fantasy? What can you change in your life now to reflect these new priorities?

_____

_____

_____

_____

_____

_____

# Gentleness Break

Before proceeding, take a gentleness break. You have already accomplished so much, and you need some time to care for yourself before going on. Here are some suggestions:

Read a story to a child.

Rediscover the fun of doodling with colored pencils or crayons.

Try a crossword puzzle.

Paddle a canoe.

Walk by a lake or stream.

Smell a flower.

Watch some birds.

Go sit in a church.

Invite a friend to take you out to dinner.

Get a massage.

Run, swim, or bike.

From this point on, there will be no more scheduled gentleness breaks. It's up to you to pace yourself and to determine when to take a break and how to spend that gentle time.

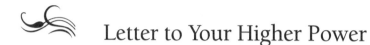 # Letter to Your Higher Power

The Second and Third Steps become very concrete when you write a letter to your Higher Power. By writing the letter, you turn your belief and trust into an active process. You will find it helpful to include in your letter how you "came to believe" and what the "decision" to turn over your will and your life means to you. Be specific about what you are turning over. Remember, the Second and Third Steps are acts of confidence or faith.

People use many different names in addressing their Higher Power, but what seems to work the best is when you make it as personal as possible.

When you have written the letter, read it out loud to your guide. We need to share our spiritual experiences with others to make sense of them.

Dear _____,

_____

_____

_____

_____

_____

_____

_____

_____

_____

_____

# Reflections
## on the
## Second and Third Steps

Trusting life comes from making some meaning of who we are, of what we are all about. When we confront shame, we become aware of emptiness, a spiritual hunger. Our attempts to fill this hunger with controlling, compulsive behaviors only lead to pain and remorse. Carl Jung was aware of this compulsive "filling of the void." He wrote to Bill Wilson, the cofounder of AA, saying that he thought alcoholism was the search for wholeness, for a "union with God."

—Merle A. Fossum and Marilyn J. Mason
*Facing Shame: Families in Recovery*

Reflect on the Fossum/Mason quote above and how you feel about the Second and Third Steps in your life.

_____

_____

_____

_____

_____

_____

_____

_____

_____

_____

The Second and Third Steps are very personal transactions and create a special intimacy when shared with others in the program. Ask the guides who have shared in your process to record their personal reactions here.

Guides: Express the trust or faith you have in the work the owner of this workbook has done.

_____

_____

_____

_____

_____

_____

_____

_____

_____

_____

_____

_____

_____

_____

Guide name: _____

Date: _____

# Step Four

Made a searching and fearless moral
inventory of ourselves.

# Step Five

Admitted to God, to ourselves, and to another human
being the exact nature of our wrongs.

With the First Step you admitted your powerlessness and vulnerability. The Second and Third Steps helped you gain the support you need from your Higher Power and other people to face the reality of addiction and coaddiction in your life. With that support you can make a fearless moral inventory and use it to examine the damage your illness has caused. This thorough self-assessment will impel you to let go of much of what keeps you in your compulsive patterns. Recovery requires giving up the old ways in which you nurtured yourself by living in the extremes. In that sense, the Fourth and Fifth Steps are a grieving process. The feelings that go into the grieving process in the Fourth and Fifth Steps include discomfort, anger, fear, shame, sadness, and loneliness. Discomfort is the outer layer of feelings, anger the second layer, and so on down to the innermost feeling of loneliness.

These feelings, which are layers of your internal self, serve as a barometer of how you feel about your behavior. They can also be a structure on which you build your moral inventory.

You will find the Fourth Step inventory to be a deeply personal experience, with each layer guiding you to a deeper relationship with yourself.

Notice, however, that the innermost layer is loneliness, in which you confront the existential reality of your aloneness and estrangement. However, the program, in its wisdom, asks you in the Fifth Step to find and share with another person the work you have done on your Fourth Step. You do not need to be alone. The program builds in more support for you at each difficult turn in your path.

The person you select to hear your Fourth Step can be someone in the program, a sponsor, or a member of the clergy. In addition to being deeply personal, the Fourth and Fifth Steps are spiritual experiences.

Before starting on your Fourth Step, set a time with the person who will hear your Fifth Step. There are several reasons for doing this. First, the Fourth Step is an awesome task and easy to put off. By making an appointment, you make a commitment to get the task done. Even if you have to reset the appointment, the focus will be on getting the Step done. Second, the person who will hear your Fifth Step may have some suggestions for you to help you in your process. Finally, you will know for sure that someone will be there for you when the path becomes difficult and painful. Again, do not forget to involve your other guides in the process as well. You do the task yourself, but you do not have to be alone. Each section will generate feelings. You do not have to wait to share them. Talk about them as they stir, not after you have figured them out.

Within each layer of feelings, you will find elements of your moral inventory that are good and positive as well as negative. As you survey the wreckage caused by your illness, you may assume that a Fourth Step focuses on all the failures, mistakes, and harm done. However, to restore integrity means to claim the successes, the goodness, the courage, and the effort as well.

Sometimes, when things seem dark, it is difficult to claim the positive in your life. If it is difficult to take credit for positive things in yourself, look at it this way. In your addiction, you probably worked hard to cover the dark side of yourself and showed only the good parts to the world. You lived between the secrets, shame, exploitation, and abuse of your hidden addict and the care, responsibility, and values of the public you. You probably even felt phony about your public self, because people did not know the real you behind the image you showed to the world. When you face the addict within you in the Fourth Step, your addiction becomes your teacher about the goodness in you. Ask yourself, Was your addict strong? Enduring? Clever? Willing to risk? Resourceful? All these are qualities your addict borrowed upon to become powerful. They are equally available to you in your recovery.

Unfortunately, many people attempt a recovery by doing the opposite of what they did in their active illness. They focus only on the bad side and bury the good. The Fourth Step presents an opportunity for you to reclaim those good parts of yourself and use them for your recovery. This is a difficult challenge, to be sure, but the result is that you get to be the real you. You don't have to have an addictive, dark side draining all your power in its secrecy. And you don't have to feel phony or insincere when you own all parts of yourself. Besides, it is much easier to face your recovery secure in the knowledge of the good things you do have to draw upon. It is the more gentle way.

The Fourth Step is a demanding and even draining experience. Pace yourself. Take several gentleness breaks. This is hard and important work, and you can take the time it deserves.

Now, proceed to your first Fourth Step inventory.

# Fourth Step Inventory: Avoiding Personal Responsibility

When taking Step Four, often the first feeling you get in touch with is discomfort. When people get uncomfortable about their behavior—especially where the potential for feeling real pain exists—they look for ways to protect themselves from the consequences of that behavior. Some of these ways are dysfunctional and self-destructive. These defensive manipulations lead us to avoid responsibility. Examples include blaming others, denial, dishonesty, intimidation, and rationalization. Sometimes you may even go to great lengths to make people in your life feel crazy. You may make up stories or act in other ways to distract or divert attention from your behavior. How have you avoided taking responsibility for your behavior? Give specific examples.

Example: Pretended Bill never told me about our appointment at school when the truth is, I forgot.

1. _____

_____

_____

2. _____

_____

_____

3. _____

_____

_____

4. _____

_____

_____

5. _____

_____

_____

6. _____

_____

_____

7. _____

_____

_____

8. _____

_____

_____

9. _____

_____

_____

10. _____

_____

_____

11. _____

_____

_____

12. _____

_____

_____

13. _____

_____

_____

14. _____

_____

_____

15. _____

_____

_____

16. _____

_____

_____

17. _____

_____

_____

18. _____

_____

_____

19. _____

_____

_____

20. _____

_____

_____

# Fourth Step Inventory: Taking Personal Responsibility

Sometimes you take responsibility for your discomfort. You can, for example, set boundaries about what you wish to talk about. Or you can express your discomfort and take responsibility for your behavior. In what ways have you clearly owned your behavior? Give specific examples.

Example: Admitted to Susan that I forgot our anniversary.

1. _____

_____

_____

2. _____

_____

_____

3. _____

_____

_____

4. _____

_____

_____

5. _____

_____

_____

6. _____

_____

_____

7. _____

_____

_____

8. _____

_____

_____

9. _____

_____

_____

10. _____

_____

_____

11. _____

_____

_____

12. _____

_____

_____

13. _____

_____

_____

14. _____

_____

_____

15. _____

_____

_____

16. _____

_____

_____

17. _____

_____

_____

18. _____

_____

_____

19. _____

_____

_____

20. _____

_____

_____

# Fourth Step Inventory: Misuse of Anger

Behind your defensive behavior there is a layer of anger. Perhaps you are angry because you got caught. Perhaps you are angry because you think people will leave you because of your behavior. You nurse grudges and resentments because you do not want to admit the damage you have done. At times you may hold on to anger so that you can stay connected to others you don't want to lose emotionally. Sometimes you might use anger to justify your addiction. In what ways have you misused your anger? Give specific examples.

Example: I used resentment toward my spouse to justify an affair.

1. _____

_____

_____

2. _____

_____

_____

3. _____

_____

_____

4. _____

_____

_____

5. _____

_____

_____


6. _____

_____

_____


7. _____

_____

_____


8. _____

_____

_____


9. _____

_____

_____


10. _____

_____

_____

11. _____

_____

_____

12. _____

_____

_____

13. _____

_____

_____

14. _____

_____

_____

15. _____

_____

_____

16. _____

_____

_____

17. _____

_____

_____

18. _____

_____

_____

19. _____

_____

_____

20. _____

_____

_____

# Fourth Step Inventory: Positive Expression of Anger

Anger empowers people to resist manipulation and exploitation. Anger can give respect and dignity in abusive situations. Within an intimate relationship, anger is inevitable. Expressing anger becomes an act of trust that the other person is important and capable of handling the anger. No relationship can survive without appropriate anger. In what ways have you been respectful and assertive with your anger? Give specific examples.

Example: I got angry with my alcoholic father when he started being cruel to my children.

1. _____

_____

_____

2. _____

_____

_____

3. _____

_____

_____

4. _____

_____

_____

5. _____

_____

_____

6. _____

_____

_____

7. _____

_____

_____

8. _____

_____

_____

9. _____

_____

_____

10. _____

_____

_____

11. _____

_____

_____

12. _____

_____

_____

13. _____

_____

_____

14. _____

_____

_____

15. _____

_____

_____

16. _____

_____

_____

17. _____

18. _____

19. _____

20. _____

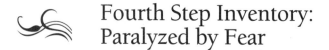

# Fourth Step Inventory: Paralyzed by Fear

Fear is the next layer of feelings. Fear can be immobilizing. When did you need to take action but did not? Make yourself vulnerable but did not? Take a risk but did not? Have you put off important tasks and discussions? In what ways have you compromised yourself by being stuck in your fear? Give specific examples.

Example: I was afraid to admit how frightened I was to leave my job—so no one understood.

1. _____
   _____
   _____

2. _____
   _____
   _____

3. _____
   _____
   _____

4. _____
   _____
   _____

5. _____

_____

_____

6. _____

_____

_____

7. _____

_____

_____

8. _____

_____

_____

9. _____

_____

_____

10. _____

_____

_____

11. _____

_____

_____

12. _____

_____

_____

13. _____

_____

_____

14. _____

_____

_____

15. _____

_____

_____

16. _____

_____

_____

17. _____

    _____

    _____

18. _____

    _____

    _____

19. _____

    _____

    _____

20. _____

    _____

    _____

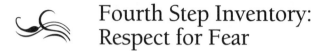

# Fourth Step Inventory: Respect for Fear

Fear serves as an important guide for your safety. Sometimes it helps you to avoid disasters and take care of yourself. When have you listened to your fear appropriately? Give specific examples.

Example: I knew it was not a good idea to date the guy I met at the airport this early in my recovery.

1. _____

   _____

   _____

2. _____

   _____

   _____

3. _____

   _____

   _____

4. _____

   _____

   _____

5. _____

_____

_____

6. _____

_____

_____

7. _____

_____

_____

8. _____

_____

_____

9. _____

_____

_____

10. _____

_____

_____

11. _____

_____

_____

12. _____

_____

_____

13. _____

_____

_____

14. _____

_____

_____

15. _____

_____

_____

16. _____

_____

_____

17. _____

_____

_____

18. _____

_____

_____

19. _____

_____

_____

20. _____

_____

_____

# Fourth Step Inventory: Taking Healthy Risks

Moments occur in which you have to set your fears aside and take significant risks. What risks have you taken for your own growth? Give specific examples.

Example: I had an idea about a new business and took the risk to try it.

1. _____

   _____

   _____

2. _____

   _____

   _____

3. _____

   _____

   _____

4. _____

   _____

   _____

5. _____

_____

_____

6. _____

_____

_____

7. _____

_____

_____

8. _____

_____

_____

9. _____

_____

_____

10. _____

_____

_____

11. _____

_____

_____

12. _____

_____

_____

13. _____

_____

_____

14. _____

_____

_____

15. _____

_____

_____

16. _____

_____

_____

17. _____

_____

_____

18. _____

_____

_____

19. _____

_____

_____

20. _____

_____

_____

# Fourth Step Inventory: Shameful Events

At an even deeper layer, addicts feel shame. You need to know where you have not lived up to your values or when you have failed to practice what you preach. Since you tell yourself that other people do not do what you did, you believe that if they found out, you would be rejected. You feel fundamentally embarrassed about yourself and unlovable. And the more shameful you feel, the more secretive you are.

A more realistic—and gentler—way of looking at your failures is to see that you are a limited human being who makes mistakes, who is lovable and forgivable. You must also remember the powerlessness and unmanageability of your illness. With these things in mind, in what ways have you not lived up to your own values? (*Suggestion:* A good guideline is to start with a list of the things you have kept secret—these are at the core of shame.) Remember, be specific.

Example: A major secret I have is . . . or I feel really bad about . . . .

1. _____

_____

_____

2. _____

_____

_____

3. _____

_____

_____

4. _____

_____

_____

5. _____

_____

_____

6. _____

_____

_____

7. _____

_____

_____

8. _____

_____

_____

9. _____

_____

_____

10.

11.

12.

13.

14.

15.

16. _____

_____

_____

17. _____

_____

_____

18. _____

_____

_____

19. _____

_____

_____

20. _____

_____

_____

# Fourth Step Inventory: Pride in Your Achievements

As a balance, you need to account for your achievements. Think of those moments when you lived up to your values or followed through on what you said you would do. Don't forget those times when you were courageous or generous and exceeded your expectations. List those times when you were intimate, vulnerable, and caring. Don't forget to include your entry into your recovery program and getting this far in the workbook! In what do you take pride? Give specific examples.

Example: I feel good about how I supported my son when he was hurt last fall.

1. _____

_____

_____

2. _____

_____

_____

3. _____

_____

_____

4. _____

_____

_____

5. _____

_____

_____

6. _____

_____

_____

7. _____

_____

_____

8. _____

_____

_____

9. _____

_____

_____

10. _____

_____

_____

11. _____

_____

_____

12. _____

_____

_____

13. _____

_____

_____

14. _____

_____

_____

15. _____

_____

_____

16. _____

_____

_____

17. _____

_____

_____

18. _____

_____

_____

19. _____

_____

_____

20. _____

_____

_____

# Fourth Step Inventory: Losses and Painful Events

Beneath shame, there is often a feeling of sadness. Many variations of sadness exist for anyone who has lived with addictive extremes. First, you grieve for all the losses: time, people, opportunities, and dreams. Second, your sorrow for those you have harmed may be quite overwhelming. Finally, there is your pain about how deeply you have been hurt by this illness. In what ways are you sad? What losses do you feel? Give specific examples in each category.

Example: I am sorry about all the times I missed being with my children.

1. _____

_____

_____

2. _____

_____

_____

3. _____

_____

_____

4. _____

_____

_____

5. _____

_____

_____

6. _____

_____

_____

7. _____

_____

_____

8. _____

_____

_____

9. _____

_____

_____

10. _____

_____

_____


I have pain about these events.

Example: I hurt because of my teacher's abuse of me.


1. _____

_____

_____


2. _____

_____

_____


3. _____

_____

_____


4. _____

_____

_____

5. _____

_____

_____

6. _____

_____

_____

7. _____

_____

_____

8. _____

_____

_____

9. _____

_____

_____

10. _____

_____

_____

# Fourth Step Inventory: Learning from Sadness

An old Buddhist saying suggests that suffering is "clinging to that which changes." Grief, sorrow, and pain simply are part of life—especially given your powerlessness over your illness and commitment to recovery. When you work through the feelings, they remain with you and add depth to who you are. You integrate new learnings. Despite the losses, your life is better than before. What gains have you made through your sadness? Give specific examples.

Example: I have learned I can live independently since my divorce.

1. _____

_____

_____

2. _____

_____

_____

3. _____

_____

_____

4. _____

_____

_____

5. _____

_____

_____

6. _____

_____

_____

7. _____

_____

_____

8. _____

_____

_____

9. _____

_____

_____

10. _____

_____

_____

11. _____

_____

_____

12. _____

_____

_____

13. _____

_____

_____

14. _____

_____

_____

15. _____

_____

_____

16. _____

_____

_____

17. _____

_____

_____

18. _____

_____

_____

19. _____

_____

_____

20. _____

_____

_____

# Fourth Step Inventory: Beliefs About Your Unworthiness

The final feeling you will reach through your Fourth Step is that of loneliness. Loneliness is created by feelings of unworthiness that separate us from others. Addicts and coaddicts have lost the most important relationship of all—the relationship with themselves. How you treat yourself becomes the lens through which you view others. Fidelity to oneself results in faithfulness to others. Integrity with oneself generates trust of others. At our core, we are alone. So each of us needs to learn to enjoy ourselves, love ourselves, trust ourselves, and care for ourselves.

*A word of caution:* This final layer may be the hardest of all to be honest about. You might find all kinds of ways to resist doing this last part thoroughly. Since your relationship with yourself is the foundation of your recovery, take time to face this part of the inventory squarely.

You need to list beliefs you have about your own unworthiness— that is, about being a "bad" person. Seeing oneself as a flawed human being is core to the belief system of all addicts and coaddicts. Some of these faulty beliefs are easily identified as not true. Others are harder to contest. List all of them you can think of.

Example: I am a deceptive person.

1. _____

_____

_____


2. _____

_____

_____

3. _____

_____

_____

4. _____

_____

_____

5. _____

_____

_____

6. _____

_____

_____

7. _____

_____

_____

8. _____

_____

_____

9. _____

10. _____

11. _____

12. _____

13. _____

14. _____

15. _____

_____

_____

16. _____

_____

_____

17. _____

_____

_____

18. _____

_____

_____

19. _____

_____

_____

20. _____

_____

_____

# Fourth Step Inventory: Self-hatred

After listing the beliefs you hold about your unworthiness, you need to be as explicit as possible about how deep the roots of your self-hatred go. As an addict, you have become an expert at beating yourself up. What things are you hardest on yourself about? Make a list of examples of self-hatred, including ways you have punished yourself, hurt yourself, put yourself down, or sold yourself out. Do not forget to include fantasies of terrible things happening to you because you somehow "deserve" them.

Example: I take projects almost to the end and don't finish them.

1. _____

_____

_____

2. _____

_____

_____

3. _____

_____

_____

4. _____

_____

_____

5. _____

_____

_____

6. _____

_____

_____

7. _____

_____

_____

8. _____

_____

_____

9. _____

_____

_____

10. _____

_____

_____

11. _____

_____

_____

12. _____

_____

_____

13. _____

_____

_____

14. _____

_____

_____

15. _____

_____

_____

16. _____

_____

_____

17. _____

_____

_____

18. _____

_____

_____

19. _____

_____

_____

20. _____

_____

_____

# Fourth Step Inventory: Self-affirmations

An affirmation is a statement about some goodness in you. Spend some time thinking about the many positive qualities you possess. How are you enjoyable, loving, caring, and trustworthy? This may also be a difficult task. Sometimes, early in recovery, good things are more evident to others than they are to you. Ask for help. When you have completed your list, you might want to read it into a tape recorder. You will have a ready-made series of affirmations when you need them.

Example: I am a person of great courage.

1. I am_____

2. I am_____

3. I am_____

4. I am_____

5. I am_____

6. I am_____

7. I am_____

8. I am_____

9. I am_____

10. I am_____

11. I am_____

12. I am_____

13. I am_____

14. I am_____

15. I am_____

16.　I am_____

17.　I am_____

18.　I am_____

19.　I am_____

20.　I am_____

21.　I am_____

22.　I am_____

23.　I am_____

24.　I am_____

25.　I am_____

26.　I am_____

27.　I am_____

28.　I am_____

29.　I am_____

30.　I am_____

# Reflections
## on the
## Fourth Step

The difficult road is the road of conversion, the conversion from loneliness into solitude. Instead of running away from our loneliness and trying to forget or deny it, we have to protect it and turn it into a fruitful solitude. To live a spiritual life, we must first find the courage to enter into the desert of our loneliness and to change it by gentle and persistent efforts into a garden of solitude. This requires not only courage, but also a strong faith. As hard as it is to believe that the dry, desolate desert can yield endless varieties of flowers, it is equally hard to imagine that our loneliness is hiding unknown beauty. The movement from loneliness to solitude, however, is the beginning of any spiritual life because it is the movement from the restless senses to the restful spirit, from the outward-reaching cravings to the inward-reaching search, from the fearful clinging to the fearless play.

—Henry Nouwen
*Reaching Out*

Read the words of Henri Nouwen above and reflect on the process of going through the layers of your Fourth Step.

Record here your reactions to facing your own loneliness.

_____

_____

_____

_____

_____

_____

_____

# Sharing Step Five: Suggestions for the Turning Point

Successful Fifth Steps come from sharing your written inventory with another person who will recognize and note the sources of greatest feeling or the places where you were stuck. As consultant as well as witness, the person who hears your Fifth Step will help you over the difficult parts of your story.

Remember also that the whole Fifth Step does not have to be done in one session. Some people who listen to Fifth Steps regularly recommend two to three sessions as opposed to a marathon event in which you share all your work at one time. Don't forget the gentleness of the path you are on.

Addicts and coaddicts often say that completing the Fifth Step was a real turning point in their recovery, that the first three Steps took on new meaning, and that they felt anchored in the program. The Fifth Step does provide special support in the person who hears your story at perhaps the most difficult point in the program. The loneliness of the Fourth Step becomes an opportunity for reaching out. A special intimacy occurs when someone accepts you even though he or she knows the very worst things about you. That experience of closeness can be duplicated as you deepen bonds with others in your life.

Spaces are provided on the following pages for you and the person you have shared your Fifth Step with to record your reactions, your feelings, and the progress you have made. Have fun with it together.

My feelings in sharing my Fifth Step

_____

_____

_____

_____

_____

_____

_____

_____

_____

_____

_____

_____

_____

_____

_____

_____

_____

_____

_____

Your name: _____

Date: _____

My feelings in hearing your Fifth Step

_____

_____

_____

_____

_____

_____

_____

_____

_____

_____

_____

_____

_____

_____

_____

_____

_____

Witness: _____

Date: _____

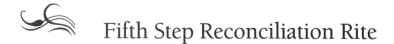 # Fifth Step Reconciliation Rite

A reader from California said he thought something was missing from the Fourth and Fifth Step exercise, but he didn't know what. When we received this gift of a reconciliation rite from an Episcopal priest, it seemed to provide the missing piece. In the priest's letter, she told us she uses it in all of the Fifth Step work that she does.

A Fifth Step is done to reestablish friendship and harmony with oneself and one's Higher Power.

- Think of one word to symbolize all you have disclosed.

- Hold out your hands to form a cup, as if someone were going to pour water into your hands.

- Say the word that represents your Fifth Step. Imagine the word resting in your hands.

- Slowly pour your Fifth Step from your hands onto the ground, as if you are letting water pour from your hands. Brush your hands, as you would to brush off sand.

- If you are doing this in the presence of your guide or your group, have them say to you, while they place a hand on you, "That which has kept you divided within yourself is gone. You are whole again."

- Repeat the phrase for yourself, "That which has kept me divided within myself is gone. I am whole again."

- Allow yourself to feel your feelings and meditate a few moments longer.

The feeling of being forgiven by a Higher Power can lead to self-forgiveness. Forgiving oneself begins the process of healing our brokenness.

Record your thoughts and feelings:

# Reflections
## on the
## Fifth Step

It strikes us when, year after year, the longed-for perfection of life does not appear, when the old compulsions reign within us as they have for decades, when despair destroys all joy and courage. Sometimes at that moment a wave of light breaks through our darkness, and it is as though a voice is saying, "You are accepted." YOU ARE ACCEPTED, accepted by that which is greater than you and the name of which you do not know. Do not ask for the name now, perhaps you will know it later. Do not try to do anything, perhaps later you will do much. Do not seek for anything, do not perform anything, do not intend anything, SIMPLY ACCEPT THE FACT THAT YOU ARE ACCEPTED.

—Paul Tillich

Read the Paul Tillich quote above and reflect on the acceptance you experienced from doing your Fifth Step.

Record your thoughts and feelings here:

# Step Six

Were entirely ready to have God remove all
these defects of character.

# Step Seven

Humbly asked Him to remove our shortcomings.

The Fourth and Fifth Steps revealed two types of shortcomings.
The first are "defects" that you originally learned as survival tools.
You developed many of your defenses as a way to cope with growing up. For example, isolation may have been the only way to cope with abuse in your family. Now that you are in recovery, you can discard dysfunctional ways of taking care of yourself. You can embrace new, healthy ways. In that sense, this stage of recovery parallels giving birth—a wondrous, painful, and at times ugly process. The exercises in this chapter are designed to help you remove your shortcomings, use a lifestyle inventory to bring your life into manageability, and develop relapse prevention tools to help you stay on the gentle path of recovery.

One thing that can stop this process is relapse—which brings us to the other type of shortcomings, the "friends" of the addict within. These friends of the addict are grandiosity, pride, willfulness, jealousy, depression, suicidal preoccupation, those aspects of yourself that combine to make you vulnerable to your addiction and coaddiction. These are the shortcomings that can return you to the compulsive spirals you were in before you entered the program. Some of these shortcomings may have helped you survive in the past, but now they are a gateway to disaster.

Several tasks can help you with the Sixth and Seventh Steps:

🎇 **Affirmations** Steps Six and Seven ask us to be willing to remove our defects. These affirmations are written to help you let go of old, familiar habits and attitudes and develop your new and positive character strengths.

🍃 **Removing Character Defects**   Helps to identify character defects. In this task, you make a list of those shortcomings you are willing to turn over to your Higher Power and the positive qualities to replace them with. For example, if dishonesty is your shortcoming, honesty is what you are working toward. Transforming weaknesses into strengths is what recovery is all about.

🍃 **Seventh Step Meditation**   Helps you visualize your life without defects and shortcomings. This exercise helps you develop a positive vision of the person you are becoming in recovery. You compose a meditation or prayer to help you remember that your Higher Power can help in this process.

🍃 **Personal Craziness Index**   Another task is to fill out a Personal Craziness Index (PCI, pronounced "picky"), a playful tool with a serious intent—to prevent relapse. The leading cause of relapse is lifestyle imbalance—being overstretched or overextended. At these times the "friends" of the addict within are immediately available.

🍃 **When Crises Occur**   Under stress it is easy to forget our new recovery behavior tools. That is why it is so important to recognize a crisis when it happens and respond with the new behaviors and inner resources you are learning about.

# Affirmations

Affirmations can help us change our behavior. We can replace unhealthy messages with messages we select. Each affirmation is written in the present—*as if* you are already accomplishing it. Even though it may not be a reality for you today, you need to "act as if." In time, telling yourself positive messages will become a familiar habit. Recovery is really a retraining program. It's about learning new ways to relate to ourselves and others. As our attitudes improve, so do our lives.

Read these affirmations to yourself or record them on tape and play them back. Pause a few seconds after each. Let the words sink deep into your consciousness. For greatest effect, repeat the exercise often.

*I enjoy taking responsibility for those things that order my life and make my life free of hassle.*

*I allow others to take responsibility for their lives.*

*I enjoy taking care of my body.*

*Exercise makes me feel healthy, strong, and happy.*

*Good nutrition allows my body to maximize its potential.*

*I do everything I need to keep myself healthy, fit, and feeling good.*

*I get the rest and relaxation I need.*

*I am financially responsible. I earn more than I spend.*

*Each day I become more organized in all areas of my life.*

*I accept that I can make mistakes and still keep trying.*

*I am grateful for a sense of humor that helps me know that I am human.*

*I meet all my obligations.   I accept only those obligations which I can meet.*

*Being on time is easy for me. I am always on time.*

*I have the courage to change.*

*I take risks that will help me grow in positive, healthy ways.*

*I value my emotions as a cherished part of me, a part to get to know, understand, and love more each day.*

*My interpersonal relationships are healthy, open, and honest.*

*I maintain the rituals of my spirituality.*

*I always allow enough time to get where I am going. I am responsible, relaxed, and organized in getting to and from my destinations.*

*I use my time, my money, my energy, and all of my resources responsibly.*

Create affirmations that are meaningful to you:

_____

_____

_____

_____

_____

_____

_____

_____

# Step Six: Removing Character Defects

Bryan, from Texas, uses *The Gentle Path* with the people he sponsors. He recognizes that addicts and coaddicts tend to feel deprived when they think of giving up something or having it removed. It is important to remember that sobriety is not about depriving oneself, but about learning how to do things differently. This exercise is designed to help you replace unhealthy defects and shortcomings with healthy behaviors.

List below your character defects or shortcomings as you see them. As you list each one, focus on the positive it can become, and list that positive quality in the parallel column.

| Defects and shortcomings I am willing to turn over | Qualities I wish to work towards |
|---|---|
| Example: Dishonesty | Example: Honesty |
| 1. _____ | 1. _____ |
| 2. _____ | 2. _____ |
| 3. _____ | 3. _____ |
| 4. _____ | 4. _____ |
| 5. _____ | 5. _____ |
| 6. _____ | 6. _____ |
| 7. _____ | 7. _____ |
| 8. _____ | 8. _____ |
| 9. _____ | 9. _____ |
| 10. _____ | 10. _____ |
| 11. _____ | 11. _____ |
| 12. _____ | 12. _____ |
| 13. _____ | 13. _____ |
| 14. _____ | 14. _____ |
| 15. _____ | 15. _____ |

# Seventh Step Meditation

Reflecting on your shortcomings, compose a prayer or meditation that you can use in times of stress to ask for help with your shortcomings. *Suggestion:* Include reminders of how desperate you were in your addiction, of your commitment to recovery, and of your powerlessness.

Lifestyle imbalance makes the addict vulnerable to relapse in the following ways.

**Feelings of entitlement**   When overextended, addicts and coaddicts seek addictive nurturing because they are so depleted. They tell themselves they are entitled and "deserve" it, rationalizing the return to self-destructive patterns.

**Increase of cravings**   When there is not enough time to take care of oneself, urges to repeat the old cycle multiply. Obsessional thinking is a relief to current stress.

**Return of denial**   In periods of imbalance, euphoric recall makes old cycles seem attractive again. Deluded thinking avoids the probable consequences of a return to previous behavior.

**Reduction of coping ability**   Overextension diminishes your ability to cope with problems. Bad decisions and poor problem solving further compound the crises in an unmanageable life.

**Participation in high-risk behaviors**   Destructive situations, persons, and events that are normally avoided become attractive under stress. The reality of unsafe behavior becomes distorted by overextension.

When you were in high school or college, you may have participated in an athletic program. Preparing for the stress of competition is called training. An athlete prepares for a stressful event (a match, game, or tournament) by observing a training program that creates extra margins of endurance and strength and that develops skills for the event. Similarly, addicts and coaddicts in a recovery program are training to participate in life. You know that you are going to experience stress, and you must prepare for that. The Twelve Steps will help you learn the necessary skills, but you also need to develop a lifestyle that builds up reserves of strength and endurance.

Think of your life as having an addiction "set point"—the point at which the imbalance leaves you vulnerable to addiction, when you are too stressed or overextended to maintain your recovery.

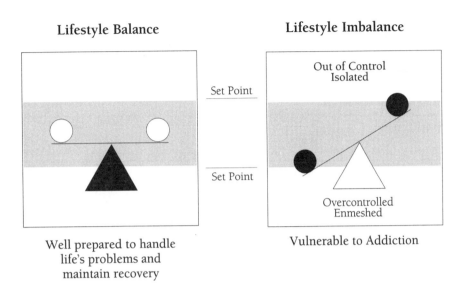

**Lifestyle Balance**

Set Point

Set Point

Well prepared to handle
life's problems and
maintain recovery

**Lifestyle Imbalance**

Out of Control
Isolated

Overcontrolled
Enmeshed

Vulnerable to Addiction

By developing a sense of what your own personal set point is, you can be alert to maintaining the balance that makes you less vulnerable to the "friends" of your addict. The PCI on page 214 will help you develop some criteria for recognizing when you have passed that point of sanity and are at risk. The PCI thus can become a set of "training" guidelines under which you train for anticipated stress. In addition, by keeping track of your own PCI for a period of time, you will get better and better at maintaining lifestyle balance and having some fun.

# Personal Craziness Index
## Part One—Preparation

The Personal Craziness Index (PCI) is based on two assumptions:

1. Craziness first appears in routine, simple behaviors that support lifestyle balance.

2. Behavioral signs will occur in patterns involving different parts of our lives. Thus, we can be caught up in issues of cosmic importance and not notice that our checking account is overdrawn. If our checking account is overdrawn, we are probably out of socks as well, because we have not done our laundry. If this pattern is pervasive, there is a risk that our lives will become emotionally bankrupt as well—cosmic issues notwithstanding.

Addicts and coaddicts are particularly vulnerable to the "insanity" of loss of reality from having neglected the basics. "Keep it simple" and "a day at a time" are not shopworn clichés, but guidelines borne out by the experience of many recovering people. The PCI helps you to remember what you need to do each day. It helps you establish good recovery habits. Without a structured process to keep you on track, "cunning and baffling," self-destructive behavior patterns will return. You'll also find the PCI helpful during periods of stress and vulnerability.

The process of creating your own PCI is designed to be as value-free as possible. Each person uses his or her own criteria to develop the index. In other words, you are asked to generate behavioral signs (or "critical incidents") which, through your own experience, you have learned to identify as danger signs or warnings that you are "losing it," "getting out of hand," or "burnt out." Thus, you will judge yourself by your own standards.

You may change the items in the index as you progress in your recovery. The following are ten areas of personal behavior suggested as sources of danger signs. Please add some of your own, if you wish.

1. **Physical Health**   The ultimate insanity is to not take care of our bodies. Without our bodies, we have nothing, yet we seem to have little

time for physical conditioning. Examples are being overweight, abusing cigarettes or caffeine, not getting regular exercise, eating junk food, getting insufficient sleep, and having a lingering sickness. When do you know that you are not taking care of your body (at least three examples)?

---

2. Transportation   How people get from place to place is often a statement about their lifestyles. Take, for example, a car owner who seldom comes to a full stop, routinely exceeds the speed limit, runs out of gas, does not check the oil, puts off needed repairs, has not cleaned out the back seat in three months, and averages three speeding tickets and ten parking tickets a year. Or the bus rider who always misses the bus, never has change, forgets his or her briefcase on the bus, and so forth. What transportation behaviors indicate that your life is getting out of control (at least three examples)?

---

3. Environment   To not have time to do your personal chores is a comment on the order of your life. Consider the home in which plants go unwatered, fish unfed, grocery supplies depleted, laundry not done or put away, cleaning neglected, dishes unwashed. What are ways in which you neglect your home or living space (at least three examples)?

---

4. Work   Chaos at work is risky for recovery. Signs of chaotic behavior are phone calls not returned within twenty-four hours, chronic lateness for appointments, being behind in promised work, an unmanageable in-basket, and "too many irons in the fire." When your life is unmanageable at work, what are your behaviors (at least three examples)?

_____

_____

_____

5. Interests   What are some positive interests besides work which give you perspective on the world? Music, reading, photography, fishing, and gardening are examples. What are you neglecting to do when you are overextended (at least three examples)?

_____

_____

_____

6. Social Life   Think of friends in your social network who constitute significant support for you and are not family or significant others. When you become isolated, alienated, or disconnected from them, what behaviors are typical of you (at least three examples)?

_____

_____

_____

7. **Family/Significant Others**   When you are disconnected from those closest to you, what is your behavior like (at least three examples)? Examples are silent, overtly hostile, and passive-aggressive.

_____

_____

_____

8. **Finances**   We handle our financial resources much as we do our emotional ones. Thus, when your checking account is unbalanced, or worse, overdrawn, or bills are overdue, or there is no cash in your pocket, or you are spending more than you earn, your financial overextension may parallel your emotional bankruptcy. List the signs that show when you are financially overextended (at least three examples).

_____

_____

_____

9. **Spiritual Life and Personal Reflection**   Spirituality can be diverse and can include such practices as meditation, yoga, and prayer. Personal reflection includes keeping a personal journal, working the Twelve Step program with daily readings, and getting therapy. What sources of routine personal reflection do you neglect when you are overextended (at least three examples)?

_____

_____

_____

10. **Other Addictions or Symptom Behaviors**   Compulsive behaviors that have negative consequences are symptomatic of your general well-being or the state of your overall recovery. When you watch inordinate amounts of TV, overeat, bite your nails—any habit you feel bad about afterward—these can be signs of burnout or possible relapse. Symptom behaviors are behaviors that are evidence of overextension, such as forgetfulness, slips of the tongue, and jealousy. What negative addiction or symptom behaviors are present when you are "on the edge" (at least three examples)?

_____

_____

_____

# Personal Craziness Index
# Part Two—Recording Your PCI

The PCI is effective only when a careful record is maintained. Recording your daily progress in conjunction with regular journal keeping will help you to keep focused on priorities that keep life manageable; work on program efforts a day at a time; expand your knowledge of personal patterns; provide a warning in periods of vulnerability to self-destructive cycles or addictive relapse.

From the thirty or more signs of personal craziness you recorded, choose the seven that are most critical for you. At the end of each day, review the list of seven key signs and count the ones you did that day, giving each behavior one point. Record your total for that day in the space provided on the chart. If you fail to record the number of points for each day, that day receives an automatic score of 7. (If you cannot even do your score, you are obviously out of balance.) At the end of the week, total your seven daily scores and make an X on the graph. Pause and reflect on where you are in your recovery. Chart your progress over a twelve-week period.

My seven key signs of personal craziness:

1. _____

2. _____

3. _____

4. _____

5. _____

6. _____

7. _____

# PCI Chart

| Day | Week | 1 | 2 | 3 | 4 | 5 | 6 | 7 | 8 | 9 | 10 | 11 | 12 |
|---|---|---|---|---|---|---|---|---|---|---|---|---|---|
| Sunday | | | | | | | | | | | | | |
| Monday | | | | | | | | | | | | | |
| Tuesday | | | | | | | | | | | | | |
| Wednesday | | | | | | | | | | | | | |
| Thursday | | | | | | | | | | | | | |
| Friday | | | | | | | | | | | | | |
| Saturday | | | | | | | | | | | | | |
| **Weekly Total** | | | | | | | | | | | | | |

# PCI Graph

50

48
Very High 46
Risk 44
42

40

38
High Risk 36
34
32

30

28
Medium Risk 26
24
22

20

18
Stable Solidity 16
14
12

10

8
Optimum 6
Health 4
2

0

# Interpretation of the PCI

A guideline for understanding your score is suggested below:

**Optimum Health**
**0–9**

Knows limits; has clear priorities; behavior congruent with values; rooted in diversity; supportive; has established a personal system; balanced, orderly, resolves crises quickly; capacity to sustain spontaneity; shows creative discipline.

**Stable Solidity**
**10–19**

Recognizes human limits; does not pretend to be more than he or she is; maintains most boundaries; well ordered; typically feels competent; feels supported; able to weather crisis.

**Medium Risk**
**20–29**

Slipping; often rushed; can't get it all in; no emotional margin for crisis; vulnerable to slip into old patterns; typically lives as if has inordinate influence over others and/or feels inadequate.

**High Risk**
**30–39**

Living in extremes (overactive or inactive); relationships abbreviated; feels and is irresponsible; constantly has reasons for not following through; lives one way, talks another; works hard to catch up.

**Very High Risk**
**40–49**

Usually pursuing self-destructive behavior; often totally into mission, cause or project; blames others for failures; seldom produces on time; controversial in community; success vs. achievement-oriented.

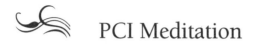 # PCI Meditation

Use the PCI as a gentle nudge to move you in the direction you want to go. As addicts and coaddicts we can get compulsive and obsessive about almost anything—self-improvement included. One coaddict who uses *The Gentle Path* described her first attempt at using the PCI. She was determined to do it right and put her life in order—once and for all. Finances had always been her greatest area of shame, so she spent two days designing a complete budget. The computerized spreadsheet listed all her income and all the bills that would be paid on each payday for the next two years. This was a good attempt on her part to put her finances in order. Unfortunately, the two days she spent doing the budget were April 14 and 15. In spending all the time on her spreadsheets, she forgot to send in her taxes. To stay on the gentle path and yet work toward your goals, here is some advice:

 

❧ **Choose to do the inventory for a specific amount of time,** such as twelve weeks, or any time period that has a specific beginning and ending. After that time, review the process and decide to extend the time or do spot-check inventories each month, each quarter, or around holidays or significant anniversary dates. The thing we know about the inventory is that it modifies behavior. If you are going to have to report on yourself every night, you will find yourself behaving in a manner that will make it comfortable for you to report on yourself.

❧ **Be patient with yourself.** To change after years of compulsive behavior is a large task. Allow yourself the luxury of making mistakes. Even taking small steps toward balance provides a sense of satisfaction.

❧ **Accept yourself.** Remember your sense of humor. Be able to laugh at some of the situations that you find yourself in, but then go on and do what you can. Accept the imperfect.

❧ **Working on your boundaries is a process—not a destination.** Set those PCI parameters as boundaries of healthy behavior—a goal to work toward. Later, when those goals have been achieved, you will want to redo the PCI and set new parameters.

❧Talk to your recovering friends about your progress and your failures. They will be your mirror to help you see when your compulsivity is getting out of control.

❧ Understand that things will change. There is as much challenge in trying to achieve balance as there was when we were constantly facing the chaos of living on the edge. The PCI is designed to give you a stable base so that when the unexpected comes up you won't be thrown off your balance.

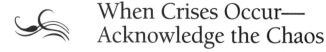

# When Crises Occur—
# Acknowledge the Chaos

Crises occur for all of us. And they seem to happen all at once, no matter how much effort we have put in. One night, flying home on a 727, I had several simultaneous crises happening. At thirty thousand feet there was little I could do. So I started to write down things I have learned about facing the inevitable crises in my life. Writing on the back of a plane ticket, I came up with fifteen action steps and five rules to remember:

## Action Steps

1. Be gentle. It's an act of trust.

2. Trust yourself. Intuition is your brain working behind your back.

3. Get help. Sometimes things are too much.

4. Create space for yourself—use environment, time, and boundaries.

5. Cocoon yourself for transformation. Surviving is not enough.

6. Embrace your antagonists. Struggle, anger, and disagreements lead to renewal.

7. Admit mistakes, including the ones no one else would know.

8. Keep focused. Grandiosity works only for the messianic.

9. Stop doing things that don't work. Trying harder only creates shame.

10. Sustain your visions. You will become your images.

11. Avoid catastrophizing. A stranglehold on reality helps you, as well as others.

12. Finish things now. Incomplete transactions make for obsession.

13. Care for your body. It is the primary spiritual act.

14. Act to contain disasters. If too late, watch.

15. Plan for surprises. Only victims are surprised.

# Rules to Remember

1. Fairness is not an issue. Reality is.

2. Fights and problems that repeat mean trouble. The issue is probably not the issue.

3. Blaming others is self-indulgent. Integrity exists only in self-responsibility.

4. Have hobbies. Competing passions maintain life balance.

5. Crises are. That's all.

# Reflections
## on the
## Sixth and Seventh Steps

Beyond a wholesome discipline,
be gentle with yourself.

You are a child of the universe, no less than the trees and the stars; you have a right to be here.

And whether or not it is clear to you, no doubt the universe is unfolding as it should.

—Desiderata

Reflect on the words above and think of what gentleness you need for yourself at this point. While you turn over your imperfections, it helps to remember your goodness and acknowledge the higher order.

Record your thoughts here:

_____

_____

_____

_____

_____

_____

_____

_____

_____

# Step Eight

Made a list of all persons we had harmed and became willing to make amends to them all.

# Step Nine

Made direct amends to such people wherever possible, except when to do so would injure them or others.

D r. Seuss explains a Ninth Step in Bartholomew and the Oobleck. We have paraphrased the story here:

They still talk about it in the kingdom of Didd as "The-Year-the-King-Got-Angry-with-the-Sky." You see, in the King's grandiosity, he had decided that he was tired of the same four things coming down from the sky: snow, fog, sunshine, and rain. He wanted something NEW to come down from the sky. And he had his way. He got what he wanted when he wanted it. He called his spooky magicians, and with magic words they made it happen. It rained oobleck! Green, gooey, molassesy stuff that stuck to everyone and wouldn't let go. The entire kingdom was paralyzed. Birds stuck to their nests, the royal musicians stuck to their instruments, the bell to warn the citizens was silenced by the green, yucky stuff. And the king sat on his throne, his royal crown stuck to his royal head.

Finally, Bartholomew Cubbins could hold his tongue no longer. "It's going to keep on falling," he shouted, "until your whole great marble palace tumbles down! So don't waste your time saying foolish magic words. YOU ought to be saying some plain, simple words!"

"*Simple* words? What do you mean, boy?"

"I mean," said Bartholomew, "this is all your fault! Now, the least you can do is say the simple words, 'I'm sorry.'"

No one had ever talked to the king like this before.

"What!" he bellowed. "ME . . . ME say 'I'm sorry!' Kings never say 'I'm sorry!'"

"But you're sitting in oobleck up to your chin. And so is everyone else in your land. And if you won't even say you're sorry, you're no sort of king at all!"

But then Bartholomew heard a great, deep sob. The old King was crying! "You're right! It is all my fault! And I am sorry! I'm awfully, awfully sorry!"

And the moment the King spoke those words, something happened.

Maybe there was magic in those simple words "I'm sorry."

Maybe there was magic in those simple words "It's all my fault."

Maybe there was, and maybe there wasn't. But they say that as soon as the old King spoke them, the sun began to shine and all the oobleck that was stuck on all the people and on all the animals of the Kingdom of Didd just simply, quietly melted away.

Saying "I'm sorry" is difficult, so we have developed several tools to help you through your Eighth and Ninth Steps.

**Record of Those Harmed and Amends Made**  A list is included to help you identify those you have harmed and how they were harmed.

**The Healer Within**  This guided imagery is designed to help you tap your inner resources for the wisdom and strength to heal yourself.

**Affirmations**  Affirmations will gently remind you of your strength for your Eighth and Ninth Step journey.

**Meditation**    This meditation will help enhance your ability to choose a new future and give you the inner discernment you need to walk the gentle path of recovery.

Besides asking for help from your Higher Power for your shortcomings, you can act on your own to mend the harm you have caused as part of your illness. In Step Eight you identify people harmed, and in Step Nine you actually make the amends necessary. When finished with Step Nine, you will have done all you can and can turn over any remaining shame and guilt. The principles of forgiveness and restitution will become an ongoing part of living your life.

Reflecting on all levels of your awareness is very important to a thorough Eighth Step. When making your list of the persons you have harmed, consider the following:

❧ **The name of the person who has been harmed.** Don't concentrate only on those people who are closest to you. Harm was done in casual relationships and acquaintanceships, as well.

❧ **Memories of harm done.** Record the specifics that you remember about the harm, including your behavior and the other person's reactions. Include facial expressions, tones of voice, circumstances, or anything that will make clear what happened.

❧ **Thoughts about the harm.** Ask yourself what you think about the situation now. Do you have reflections or interpretations about the harm?

❧ **Feelings about the harm.** Acknowledge the pain, anger, shame, guilt, and fear that you have about the situation now. Also ask yourself what feelings you have about attempting to repair the damage.

❧ **Intentions you now have.** Perhaps the hardest part is to determine what you hope to accomplish by doing some repair work. Sometimes our intentions are not helpful. If, for example, your intent is to look good to others, you probably need to take a longer look at your motives.

❧ **Amends you can make for the harm caused.** Name specific actions that will make up for what happened. Sometimes that may mean simply saying "I'm sorry." You will find some situations for which nothing can be done. For example, you have no idea how to reach someone, and the only amend you can make is to live your life differently. In some situations, further contact might cause further harm. At least you will be able to integrate that fact into your self-awareness. At the conclusion, you will have a list of all the amends you are willing to make. You will also have some blank spaces when it comes to amends.

As you can see, this will be a lengthy, difficult, soul-searching process that requires creativity and courage. Your guides can be important here. By reviewing your process as you go along, your guides can help you stay in reality. Their reactions to certain events may differ from yours, or they may challenge your intentions or suggest alternative actions. Remember, these amends do not have to be done all at once. You deserve time to think and to feel the process through. Again, gentleness is your goal.

The next several pages provide a worksheet for you to use. On the far right is a space labeled "Date." As you make each amend, record the date it was completed. By updating the column, you will know exactly where you are on your Ninth Step. Entering the dates will remind you to call your guides and update them as well.

# Record of Those Harmed and Amends Made

**Person:**

Memories of Harm

Thoughts

Feelings

Intentions

Amends

**Date:**

# Record of Those Harmed and Amends Made *(continued)*

**Person:** _____

Memories of Harm _____

_____

_____

_____

Thoughts _____

_____

_____

_____

Feelings _____

_____

_____

_____

Intentions _____

_____

_____

_____

Amends _____

_____

_____

**Date:** _____

# Record of Those Harmed and Amends Made *(continued)*

**Person:** _____

Memories of Harm _____

_____

_____

_____

Thoughts _____

_____

_____

_____

Feelings _____

_____

_____

_____

Intentions _____

_____

_____

_____

Amends _____

_____

_____

**Date:** _____

# Record of Those Harmed and Amends Made *(continued)*

**Person:**

Memories of Harm

Thoughts

Feelings

Intentions

Amends

**Date:**

# Record of Those Harmed and Amends Made *(continued)*

**Person:** _____

Memories of Harm _____

_____

_____

_____

Thoughts _____

_____

_____

_____

Feelings _____

_____

_____

_____

Intentions _____

_____

_____

_____

Amends _____

_____

_____

**Date:** _____

# Record of Those Harmed and Amends Made *(continued)*

**Person:**

Memories of Harm

Thoughts

Feelings

Intentions

Amends

**Date:**

# The Healer Within

We all have untapped reserves of energy within us. We can learn to draw upon that strength. In non-Western cultures, the Healer is an integrating force in the life of its community and individuals. These Healers have several responsibilities, not just the healing of the sick. If we look at their responsibilities and then mirror them within ourselves, we may draw upon healing forces we did not know we possessed. We all have a Healer Within. We also have a Child Within that needs to be cared for, guided, and nurtured so that it can just be. Read the following descriptions of what Healers do, what your Healer Within does, and what your Child Within needs.

## What Healers do

Healers mobilize belief. They tap those sources of energy that have not been available to individuals by themselves.

> *What your Healer Within does*
> Learns to trust intuition. Believes in self.

> *What your Child Within does*
> Preserves its innocence.

## What Healers do

Healers release energy. With enthusiasm or charisma they are a catalyst and motivating force.

> *What your Healer Within does*
> Gathers energy to itself to mobilize.

> *What your Child Within does*
> Releases the energy in play.

## What Healers do

They make sense out of the chaos.

> *What your Healer Within does*
> Protects itself from the chaos by creating boundaries.
>
> *What your Child Within does*
> Lives in safety.

## What Healers do

Healers provide wisdom.

> *What your Healer Within does*
> Accesses your own wisdom. Some ways to do this are journaling, meditating, and imaging solutions.
>
> *What your Child Within does*
> Seeks guidance.

## What Healers do

They convene community. They bind others in community by uniting people with a feeling of belonging.

> *What your Healer Within does*
> Builds community by organizing, participating, or reaching out.
>
> *What your Child Within does*
> Needs to belong to a community.

## What Healers do

Healers use symbols and metaphors to teach and help others understand.

> *What your Healer Within does*
> Discovers symbols and metaphors. Makes the connections and understands the analogies.
>
> *What your Inner Child does*
> Inherits the metaphors, symbols, and understanding.

## What Healers do

Healers are the storytellers. By preserving traditions, they anchor individuals in their community and place in history.

> *What your Healer Within does*
> Acknowledges your story, your epoch, and your place in history.

> *What your Child Within does*
> Gets to be the hero of the story.

## What Healers do

Healers provide care.

> *What your Healer Within does*
> Nurtures the self.

> *What your Child Within does*
> Accepts nurturing.

## What Healers do

Healers channel the spiritual.

> *What your Healer Within does*
> Accesses the spiritual—the presence of God within.

> *What your Child Within does*
> Is present to the world and to emotions. Being present is a spiritual act.

## What Healers do

Healers lead the collective process.

> *What your Healer Within does*
> Becomes a partner, a participant, in the process.

> *What your Child Within does*
> Is allowed to be vulnerable and surrender to the process.

## What Healers do

Often Healers are wounded themselves. Healing their own brokenness gave them the wisdom to heal others.

> *What your Healer Within does*
> Attends and heals your wounds and brokenness.

> *What your Child Within does*
> Is allowed to acknowledge suffering and admit pain.

## What Healers do

Healers witness the truth.

> *What your Healer Within does*
> Discerns truth. Recognizes falsehood for what it is.

> *What your Child Within does*
> Speaks and lives the truth.

When we call upon the Healer Within, we have a powerful resource for healing our Child Within. The Healer Within becomes a protector and champion to our Child Within. It allows the Child Within to preserve its innocence. It allows it to play, feel safe, seek guidance, and accept the desire to belong to its community. The Child Within inherits the heroic epics, stories, and metaphors that interpret inner chaos and provide wisdom. The Healer Within allows the Child to trust in its own spirituality by being present to the world, acknowledging suffering and pain, and speaking the truth. The Healer Within allows the Child Within to accept nurturing and not fear being vulnerable.

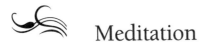 # Meditation

The following meditation is designed to help you visualize your Healer Within for the Child Within. You may choose to read it into a tape recorder and play it back, or have someone read it aloud to you. Pause for ten to fifteen seconds where indicated, or turn off the tape recorder, before continuing.

*Find a nice, comfortable position.*

*If you are feeling anything emotionally distressing, picture yourself putting it in a box and setting it aside until the meditation is over. [pause]*

*Get in touch with your own bodily rhythms, your breathing, your heart rate. With each breath you take, each beat of your heart, you are participating in the larger rhythms of the universe. Each of those beats, each of those rhythms, has a sacredness to it because it is part of the forces of the universe. [pause]*

*Imagine that you are lying in a meadow on a summer day. You can feel the sun on your body. You feel very, very peaceful. You can hear the birds singing, smell the flowers and the grasses of the field. [pause]*

*You feel beckoned, as if you are being asked to go somewhere. You hear a voice calling you. You gently sit up. You look around. At the end of the meadow is a road. You know that road is where you need to go. You get up and walk to the road at the edge of the meadow. You walk down the road. As you walk, you come around the corner to a lake where there is a beach. There a child is playing in the sand on the beach. [pause]*

*As you approach, you see something familiar about that child. You leave the road. As you come closer, you see that the child is you at the age of five. This is what you looked like. This is who you were at the age of five. You get down on your knees and look at the child at the child's level, and you ask the child how the child is doing.*

*What does the child say to you? [pause]*

*Walk with the child. Invite the child to come along with you on your journey. Reach out and offer the child your hand. Ask the child to join you. The two of you leave the beach and go on down the road. [pause]*

*As you walk down the road, you come to some large hills at the base of a mountain. Up on one of the hills is a large, sanctuary-like building. You and the child approach the building. There is a long flight of stairs in front of the building. As the two of you come to the flight of stairs, a man and a woman walk out. They are so peaceful looking. They say, "Come, we have been waiting for you." You and the child walk up the stairs, and the man and the woman each take your hands and say, "We're so glad you are here."*

*Now they invite you in. They say to you, "We want to take you to what we call the room of vision." They guide you into a room with multicolored glass in the ceiling and skylights. There is no furniture, but a soft, spongy floor and four walls. [pause]*

*Your guides ask you to sit down. They explain to you that the room of visions is a way to have windows into your life.*

*The woman guide turns to your child and asks, "What is hurting you?" [pause] "How do you hurt right now?" [pause]*

*What does your child say to the woman right now? [pause]*

*The man turns to you and asks, "What is troubling you?" [pause]*

*What do you say to the man? [pause]*

Then the woman explains, "We brought you here because we know you are troubled and we believe that there are things you already know that can help. Each wall to this room contains a vision. Two of the walls have visions of your future. Let's look at the first one."

The wall dissolves and there is an image of your future. You are watching you in your own future. What is this image about? [pause] What is happening in your future? [pause] What do you see? [pause] How do you react to this vision of the future? [pause] Look at your child. How is your child reacting to this vision from the future? [pause] The man says to you, "Now, remember, you can choose whether you want this in your future. Make a decision."

Look at your child. Is the child comfortable? [pause] Look at the future. Do you want this as part of your future? [pause] Make your decision and, as you decide, watch as the wall goes blank.

The guides then point to another wall. It dissolves and another vision comes out of your future. What is happening in this vision? [pause] What are you doing? [pause] Who are you with? [pause] How does it look like you are feeling in this future? [pause] How do you feel watching it? [pause] How does your child feel? [pause] Look at your child. How is your child reacting to it? [pause]

The woman says to you, "Now, again you can make a decision. Is this what you want?" [pause] "Is this what you want in your future?" [pause] "Choose." As you make your decision, the wall becomes opaque again. [pause]

The man guide says, "Behind the third wall are gifts. The child is to go first." The wall dissolves, and there is a gift waiting there for the child. What is the gift? [pause] "This is a spiritual gift," the man says. "Have your child go and get the gift and then come back and sit down on the soft, warm floor."

As you look up, your other guide says, "There is a gift in there for you, a spiritual gift. Let it be a symbol for you." What is the gift? [pause] What does it look like? [pause] What characteristics does it have? [pause] Get up and walk over to the gift. Pick it up and bring it back.

Behind the fourth wall, your guide says, "Picture an animal that you think is like you. An animal that can have special significance." Your child goes first. What animal appears for your child? [pause] Your guide asks, "How are you like this animal?" [pause] "In what ways are you like this animal?" [pause]

Now it is your turn. What animal fits for you? [pause] The wall dissolves and you can picture that animal. What is it like? [pause] How are you like that animal? [pause] What characteristics does it have that are like you? [pause]

Your guide says, "Let these animals serve as symbols for you of what you are about. Learn about them. Study them. They will teach you what you need to know."

You and your guides rise and you walk out of the building, into a garden, and down the stairs. You sit down next to your child. Spend a little time now, talking to that child. What do the Healers say to that child? [pause] What did you learn? [pause] How can you use the gifts? [pause] What about the future? Talk to the child. [pause]

As you finish the conversation, take the child's hand and walk back to the beach.

Promise your child that you will let your child play, but that you will leave now. Whenever that child needs you, you will be back. Promise that the Healer Within you will always be there for the child. [pause]

As you walk away, back towards the meadow, you are aware that something has shifted. Something will never be the same. You feel steadier. You trust yourself. You are more peaceful. Sturdier. As you lay down in the meadow, you can feel the presence of the moment, *how you blend into the earth, embracing it. You decide to rest, and you go to sleep.*

*When you are ready to finish the fantasy, awake and arise slowly and peacefully. Hold onto the feelings of your imagery.*

Healing is a matter of nurture, comfort, story, images, and personal connection. There are times when the child needs the healer, but there are also times when the healer needs the playfulness of the child. Metaphors are another way to get at your reality. If someone told you to play more, that you have the capability, it wouldn't be very effective. But if you can image yourself as an animal playing, or the child playing, it becomes believable to you on a conscious level. The visualization you just completed is a metaphor. Describe your images and thoughts during the process.

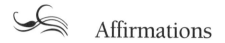 # Affirmations

Affirmations can help us change our behavior. We can replace unhealthy messages that we did not choose with healthy messages we select. Each affirmation is written in the present—as if you are already accomplishing it. Even though it may not be a reality for you today, you need to "act as if." It may be difficult, but think of it as planting a garden with possibilities that will bloom with wonderful realities.

Select from the list the affirmations that have meaning for you, and add some of your own. Read them each day or as you need them. Place the list of affirmations on your mirror and repeat them while you are shaving or putting on your makeup. Keep a copy in the car to repeat while commuting, or record them on a tape and let the tape tell them to you right before you fall asleep.

*I take responsibility for my part in my interpersonal relationships.*

*I am ruthlessly honest in determining my part in a relationship that has been damaged.*

*I can restore my own integrity by being willing to change, to disclose secrets, create new boundaries, be discerning in understanding systems, be willing to finish things, be open to new relationships and take responsibility.*

*I am willing to look honestly at my sexual relationships. I acknowledge that as a sexual being, my sexuality is an integral part of my recovery. I apply honesty and spirituality to healing the sexual part of my life.*

*I am open to the spiritual healing of the amends process. Whatever the outcome of my attempt, I will take pride in trying to make my amend.*

*I ask for guidance in choosing whether to make an amend. With this guidance, I will not hurt myself or anyone further.*

*I am open to the lessons that I can learn from making amends, and I am grateful for them.*

# Reflections
## on the
## Eighth and Ninth Steps

If we are painstaking about this phase of our development, we are halfway through. We are going to know a new freedom and a new happiness. We will not regret the past or wish to shut the door on it. We will comprehend the word serenity and we will know peace. No matter how far down the scale we have gone, we will see how our experience can benefit others. That feeling of uselessness and self-pity will disappear. We will lose interest in selfish things and gain interest in our fellows. Self-seeking will slip away. Our whole attitude and outlook upon life will change. Fear of people and of economic insecurity will leave us. We will intuitively know how to handle situations that used to baffle us. We will suddenly realize that God is doing for us what we could not do for ourselves.

Alcoholics Anonymous—The "Big Book"

These are the famous promises of the program. Reflect on completing your Eighth and Ninth Steps.

Guides: What examples of the promises at work do you see in the life of this workbook owner?

Record your reactions here:

_____

_____

_____

_____

_____

_____

_____

_____

_____

_____

_____

_____

_____

_____

_____

_____

_____

_____

Guide name: _____

Date: _____

# Step Ten

### Continued to take personal inventory and when we were wrong promptly admitted it.

Step Ten asks you to integrate the program principles of honesty and spiritual exploration into your daily life. By now you will have noticed that the program asks you at different points to be a list maker. Making lists becomes one way for you to develop personal awareness. Daily monitoring of the realities of your strengths and limitations plus a willingness to acknowledge your failings and successes is the surest path to sanity. From the beginning of this workbook we have emphasized balance, focus, and self-responsibility. Applying those concepts to Step Ten we see

**Balance**   Acknowledging strengths and limitations.

**Focus**   Taking a daily personal inventory.

**Self-responsibility**   Acknowledging successes and failures promptly.

This commitment to integrity lays the foundation for active spirituality. Conversely, such rigorous ongoing self-examination can be sustained only with a strong spiritual base—Step Eleven. The combination of the two becomes a way of life for program people. The spiritual component grows through daily readings, meditation, prayer, and journal writing.

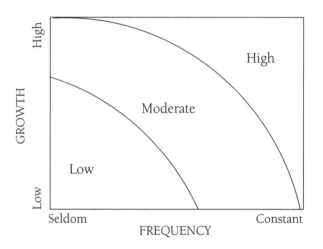

Figure 2   Impact of Recovery

By maintaining this balance, focus, and self-responsibility, recovering people create an "open system" that grows and adapts. This contrasts with the "closed" (rigid, judgmental) and the chaotic (random, purposeless) systems of addiction and coaddiction. Making lists, doing Step work, keeping a journal, attending workshops, and participating in therapy and treatment are all examples of recovery activities that help expand our awareness and growth. A growing system stays in balance.

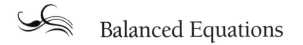 Balanced Equations

## A Ten-Day Exercise for Steps Ten and Eleven

In the following exercise, ten equations are provided that represent the essential, but delicate, balance we all need in our lives. The first equation, the happiness equation, is taken from Dan Milan's *Way of the Peaceful Warrior,* which served as the inspiration for the exercise. These equations are illustrations of the relative components of these key recovery issues:

Happiness

Growth

Serenity

Peace of mind

Reality

Achievement

Intimacy

Productivity

Health

Spirituality

Use each equation as a daily meditation upon imbalances in your life. Record your reflections, and then compose a prayer for each day, a prayer that helps you strike a balance. Stay in the moment. Describe thoughts and feelings that are present for you today.

At the end of the ten days, have a discussion with your guides about what process you would like to develop and use to maintain your conscious contact with God. Spirituality is fundamentally a personal and dynamic process. In addition to daily meditation and prayer, your plan to keep your connection to your Higher Power may include any practices—from helping others to sitting by a stream—that work for you. The exercises in the next section can help you achieve the balance you need to stay spiritually centered.

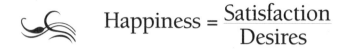 Happiness = $\dfrac{\text{Satisfaction}}{\text{Desires}}$

## Day One

Happiness exists when what you want is matched by what you have. If your desires are few, they are easy to satisfy.

Are you so obsessed with what you do not have that you miss what you have now? Are your desires so intense that you always have to be striving for more to satisfy them?

## Reflection

Prayer

_____

_____

_____

_____

_____

_____

_____

_____

_____

_____

_____

_____

_____

_____

_____

_____

_____

_____

_____

_____

Growth = $\dfrac{\text{Change}}{\text{Stability}}$

## Day Two

Systems need to change or they die. Change is an essential ingredient to growth. Change without a stable foundation, however, leads to chaos. Any recovery program has elements of change as well as elements of stability.

Do you have a stable foundation to support your growth? Are you afraid to risk change, remaining stuck where you are?

## Reflection

_____

_____

_____

_____

_____

_____

_____

_____

_____

_____

_____

_____

Prayer

_____

_____

_____

_____

_____

_____

_____

_____

_____

_____

_____

_____

_____

_____

_____

_____

_____

_____

_____

_____

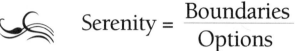 Serenity = $\dfrac{\text{Boundaries}}{\text{Options}}$

## Day Three

Addicts and coaddicts live in the extremes, which means they can take any option to an excess. Imposing limits in the form of boundaries creates balance. The Serenity Prayer epitomizes this principle by praying for courage "to change the things I can."

Do you pursue all your possibilities without any limits? Are you too caring, too helpful, too involved, too committed, too generous?

## Reflection

_____

_____

_____

_____

_____

_____

_____

_____

_____

_____

_____

_____

_____

_____

# Prayer

_____

_____

_____

_____

_____

_____

_____

_____

_____

_____

_____

_____

_____

_____

_____

_____

_____

_____

_____

_____

Peace of Mind = $\dfrac{\text{Known to Others}}{\text{Known to Self}}$

## Day Four

Anxiety originates in secrets about yourself that others do not know. Worry about others discovering the truth destroys your peace of mind. When there are others in your life who know all there is to know, you can be peaceful and stop living in terror of another abandonment.

Are you living in fear because of untold secrets? Have you lied to people because you wanted to avoid conflict or hurting someone? Do you have friends you can confide your fear to?

### Reflection

---

# Prayer

Reality = $\dfrac{\text{Light Side}}{\text{Dark Side}}$

## Day Five

Reality is acknowledging both your strengths and your weaknesses. To focus only on your failures distorts reality. To see only the successes equally blurs your vision. Both need to be full—not partially—acknowledged and accepted.

Do you have more difficulty admitting strengths or weaknesses? Do you fully admit that you have both?

## Reflection

Prayer

_____

_____

_____

_____

_____

_____

_____

_____

_____

_____

_____

_____

_____

_____

_____

_____

_____

_____

_____

_____

_____

_____

_____

Achievement = $\dfrac{\text{Vision}}{\text{Plan}}$

## Day Six

Genuine achievement combines both an image of what needs to be done and a concrete plan of action to get the tasks done. A plan without vision goes nowhere. A vision without concrete action never becomes reality. Part of thinking "a day at a time" is to break a dream down into little pieces that can be done a "piece" at a time.

Do you procrastinate about taking action on your ideas? Do you think about what you want to do before you act? Do you break big dreams into daily, doable pieces?

## Reflection

_____

_____

_____

_____

_____

_____

_____

_____

_____

_____

_____

_____

_____

_____

# Prayer

_____

_____

_____

_____

_____

_____

_____

_____

_____

_____

_____

_____

_____

_____

_____

_____

_____

_____

_____

_____

_____

_____

Intimacy = $\dfrac{\text{Fidelity to Others}}{\text{Fidelity to Self}}$

## Day Seven

Ultimately, intimacy exists because of trust. When fidelity to yourself matches faithfulness to others, trust occurs. People who report clearly their own needs, boundaries, and feelings are trustworthy. You can predict—or trust—what they will do. If you are accountable to others, people will feel safe being close to you.

Do you compromise yourself or give in too easily and then get mad? Do you say yes when you really want to say no? Do you follow through on your promises? Can people trust you enough to be intimate?

## Reflection

_____

_____

_____

_____

_____

_____

_____

_____

_____

_____

_____

Prayer

_____

_____

_____

_____

_____

_____

_____

_____

_____

_____

_____

_____

_____

_____

_____

_____

_____

_____

_____

_____

_____

_____

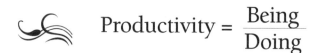 Productivity = $\dfrac{\text{Being}}{\text{Doing}}$

## Day Eight

Truly productive people take time to re-create themselves by doing nothing. Stopping to enjoy all that is around you is essential to renewing your energy. What you do needs to be matched by times of simply being.

Do you stop to smell the flowers? Do you have "busy" vacations? Do you have daily downtime? Do you take time to be quiet? Are you meditating too much and not accomplishing anything concrete?

## Reflection

Prayer

_____

_____

_____

_____

_____

_____

_____

_____

_____

_____

_____

_____

_____

_____

_____

_____

_____

_____

_____

_____

_____

_____

Health = $\dfrac{\text{Awareness}}{\text{Practice}}$

## Day Nine

As a recovering person, you need to take greater responsibility for your health. This means that you need to learn about it and develop your awareness. Your awareness must be matched by action. Do you do what you know you should?

Are there aspects of your own health you need to know more about? Do you take care of yourself physically and respect your body? Are you doing what you need to?

## Reflection

_____

_____

_____

_____

_____

_____

_____

_____

_____

_____

_____

_____

Prayer

_____

_____

_____

_____

_____

_____

_____

_____

_____

_____

_____

_____

_____

_____

_____

_____

_____

_____

_____

_____

_____

_____

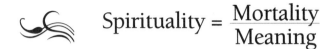

# Spirituality = $\dfrac{\text{Mortality}}{\text{Meaning}}$

## Day Ten

Spirituality starts with understanding your own human limitations, beginning with your mortality. Given those limits, you need to explore what meaning they have for you. Philosophical speculation without the reality of your human limits has no foundation and quickly becomes irrelevant. Daily life becomes pointless and without a sense of higher purpose.

Do you live each day as if it were your last? Did you find time today to address your priorities?

## Reflection

_____

_____

_____

_____

_____

_____

_____

_____

_____

_____

_____

_____

_____

_____

Prayer

_____

_____

_____

_____

_____

_____

_____

_____

_____

_____

_____

_____

_____

_____

_____

_____

_____

_____

_____

_____

# Daily Tenth Step Inventory

Using the equations as reminders, each day mentally review these areas of your life as a Tenth Step inventory.

🍃 **Happiness**  Did you balance satisfaction with desires?

🍃 **Growth**  Did you balance your need for stability with what is healthy, new, and different?

🍃 **Serenity**  Did you balance your possibilities with your limitations?

🍃 **Peace of Mind**  Did you take the risk to not keep secrets from those you trust?

🍃 **Reality**  Did you list the strengths and weaknesses that you demonstrated today?

🍃 **Achievement**  Did you plan or act on your vision for yourself today?

🍃 **Intimacy**  Did you find balance between your boundaries and accountability to others?

🍃 **Productivity**  Was there balance between what you accomplished and moments of peace for you today?

🍃 **Health**  What did you do today to take care of your body?

🍃 **Spirituality**  What action did you take today to touch a sense of your higher purpose and your own humanity?

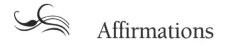 # Affirmations

Affirmations help us change our behavior. Read the following into a tape recorder and listen to the person you are now and are becoming. Pause a few seconds between each affirmation.

*I create my own happiness by allocating my resources to achieve those things that give me satisfaction.*

*I have a firm foundation of stability in several areas of my life that allows me to positively change to continue my growth in recovery.*

*The options I select and the boundaries I establish give me serenity.*

*My peace of mind comes from trusting my intimate circle with my reality.*

*I accept my strengths and weaknesses, my good and bad choices that help me through the gray of reality.*

*Vision creates the purpose and direction for my life. I achieve my purpose with planning and execution—one piece at a time.*

*Trust in myself and in others allows me intimacy.*

*My productivity is maximized when I accomplish tasks and spend time re-creating myself.*

*I perform healthful practices out of respect and reverence for my body's needs.*

*Each moment in my day holds an opportunity to give my life higher meaning by how I choose to live it.*

Create affirmations that are meaningful to you:

_____

_____

_____

# Reflections
## on the
### Tenth and Eleventh Steps

We must always hold truth, as best we can determine it, to be more important, more vital to our self-interest, than our comfort. Conversely, we must always consider our personal discomfort relatively unimportant and, indeed, even welcome it in the service or the search for truth. Mental health is an ongoing process of dedication to reality at all costs...What does a life of total dedication to truth mean? It means, first of all, a life of continuous and never ending stringent self-examination.

—M. Scott Peck, M.D.
*The Road Less Traveled*

Reflect on the words of Scott Peck and think of your daily meditation and prayer practices. Do they help you maintain conscious contact with your Higher Power? Do they help you with your ongoing personal inventory?

Guides: What do you see happening on a daily basis in the life of this workbook owner?

Share your insights, feelings, and suggestions here:

_____

_____

_____

_____

_____

_____

_____

_____

_____

_____

_____

_____

_____

_____

_____

_____

_____

Guide name: _____

Date: _____

# Step Eleven

Sought through prayer and meditation to
improve our conscious contact with God *as we
understood Him*, praying only for knowledge of His will
for us and the power to carry that out.

Spiritual renewal has many forms. Throughout the *Gentle Path* series
we have suggested a variety of strategies and daily activities. Those
suggestions certainly fit the intention of Step Eleven. Sometimes we
need to make an extraordinary effort, especially if we are in need of
direction in our lives. Spirituality is simply another level of "knowing" or
finding. Often this takes the form of a journey or quest. To undertake
such a spiritual quest, you will need to make special preparations. Here
are suggestions for what you might need:

**A dream journal.** Buy yourself a book with blank pages. As you
plan and prepare for this quest, keep a log of all dreams you remember,
even if they are only fragments. If you have trouble remembering your
dreams, keep a tape recorder by your bed. Transcribe the dreams in the
morning. Record the day, the dream, and the feelings you had as part of
the dream. Dreams bear important messages from within ourselves.
While on your quest, your dream log may become very important to
you.

**A seeking place.** Select a time when you will be undisturbed, such
as during a weekend, series of weekends, week, month—whatever you
can manage to dedicate to your spiritual quest. This time should be
when you can lay daily demands aside and not be distracted by family,
friends, job, or other factors.

**A guiding metaphor.** Look for an analogy or metaphor for this
time of your life. Survivors of child abuse, for example, often use the turtle. They notice how the ways of the turtle can be helpful. Turtles are
survivors of eons of evolution; they evolved a tough shell to protect vul-

nerable parts; they pursue a deliberate pace on land but allow themselves grace in the open seas; and they know how to pull in to avoid harm. Find a metaphor or analogy that can help you think about this time.

**A collection of sacred things.** Native Americans have the concept of a medicine bundle. Recovering people use the concept of a "God box." Whatever term you use, gather together things of special significance to you that symbolize empowered moments of your life. Program medallions, sponsor gifts—collect anything that will help you connect with your own spiritual roots.

**A spiritual mentor.** Based upon their own experience, a spiritual director or holy person can help you. Whether it be the exercises of St. Ignatius or the Vision Quest of the Sioux, holy persons help prepare you for the quest. They support you during the experience. They debrief you later to help you understand your experiences. They are special guides for this time.

Usually a quest takes months of preparation and lots of coaching from the spiritual mentor. Sometimes there are readings to be done, information to be gathered, or special materials to be found. There is no magic in this preparation. It is simply preparing yourself.

During the actual quest, take care to journal your experiences. Share them only with your spiritual guide. Allow time from daily living with your guide to process this retreat. We have included a planning sheet for you to think about your quest. We have provided space for your guide to memorialize whatever reactions he or she had.

Blessings on your effort!

# Spiritual Quest Planning Sheet

Complete the following in preparation for your quest.

1.  What is the "seeking place" you will use?

_____

_____

2.  When is your "seeking time?"

_____

_____

3.  What metaphors will you use?

_____

_____

4.  What special, sacred thing do you wish to bring with you?

_____

5.  Who will serve as your spiritual mentor?

_____

6.  What special instructions does your spiritual mentor suggest?

_____

_____

_____

# Spiritual Quest Debriefing

This sheet is intended for spiritual guides to share reactions and observations of those they have supported in making a spiritual quest. Write, in a letter form, affirming the quest and any special efforts and gains this person has made because of the experience. Summarize what learnings you see as most important for future action. Remember that this letter is a very important part of the workbook. It serves as a "meaning anchor" to deepen this person's spiritual experience and as a touchstone for the person's continuing journey in recovery.

Date: _____

Dear _____ ,

_____

_____

_____

_____

_____

_____

_____

_____

_____

_____

_____

_____

_____

_____

_____

_____

# Step Twelve

Having had a spiritual awakening as a result of these steps, we tried to carry this message to alcoholics, and to practice these principles in all our affairs.

As this edition of *The Gentle Path* is being prepared, a community of fifty men is struggling with denial and acceptance, seeking sobriety and a definition of spirituality that they can understand, and a chance—perhaps only a slim one—not to die from the side effects of their drug and sexual addiction. These men live in a community called Jericho. Like its namesake, Jericho has walls—walls that keep 4,500 other prisoners out. Jericho is an addiction and drug rehabilitation center in a Pennsylvania prison. Because of the rampant drug and sex addiction there, AIDS is also widespread. For these men, becoming— and staying—clean and sober literally means they may not have to die in prison from AIDS.

Jericho is only one of the millions of reasons Twelve Step work is so important. We may never really know if a talk we give at an open meeting or in a detox center actually changed someone's life. We may not always see the impact we make on the person we sponsor or on how that person's experience helps someone else. Sharing your recovery with others is like making a ripple in a lake. Maybe one of the people you touch, who then touches another, will make a difference in someone's sobriety.

Oh, yes, one of the million reasons to do Twelve Step work is so you stay sober.

Helping others is a significant part of the program, and there are many ways the program gets passed on. When you live the program and share it with others, you are carrying the message, especially when you sponsor new members. In practicing the Twelfth Step you will find that

&❧ By witnessing to others, your appreciation of the program and the program's impact on your life deepens.

&❧ By hearing the stories of new members, you are reminded of where you were when you started.

ﻌ By modeling to others, you become aware that you need to practice what you preach.

ﻌ By giving to others, you develop bonds with new people who really need you.

ﻌ By helping others, you give what you have received.

ﻌ By supporting new beginnings, you revitalize your own efforts.

Being a sponsor sounds intimidating, but there are only a few things you need to do:

ﻌ Work hard to understand the whole story of the person you are sponsoring.

ﻌ Give emotional support to the person you are sponsoring during those difficult times.

ﻌ Help the person you are sponsoring to focus on the basics of your particular program.

ﻌ Help the person you are sponsoring to focus on the Steps of the program.

In your relationships with those you sponsor, you will be finding good things about them that they overlook. (Remember when all you could find to report to your sponsor was the latest disaster?) You will work hard to help new members see what it is they are doing right. Addicts and coaddicts, by definition, see only the bad in themselves. Perhaps the most priceless gifts a sponsor can give are those beginning affirmations.

As a sponsor, you serve as a special role model. How you work your program will have a significant impact on those you help. To bolster your confidence, have your guides share their reactions to your being a sponsor using the space provided on page 288.

You also need to be very clear about your own definition of sobriety. To review that again will help you be more clear with the person you are sponsoring. No doubt your understanding of your sobriety has evolved since those early days when you told the group what you would not do. The sobriety worksheet provided reflects the old Buddhist axiom that wisdom is being able to say yes as well as no. In sobriety terms, this means that recovery is more than abstinence from self-destructive behavior. It is also a positive statement about what you embrace.

Much of this has probably been clear to you for some time, but recording and discussing your personal standards of sobriety with your own guides will be helpful to you and those you are about to help.

Remember, your path is gentle. You can get help in learning to help others. Your Higher Power will be with you.

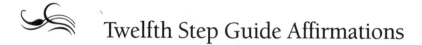

# Twelfth Step Guide Affirmations

The purpose of this page is for your guides to affirm you and your suitability to help others on the gentle path.

*Note to guides and friends:* As you list affirmations, the more specific you can be, the more helpful the affirmations will be.

Example: You are are one of the best listeners I know. —*S.K.*

1. _____

   _____

2. _____

   _____

3. _____

   _____

4. _____

   _____

5. _____

   _____

6. _____

   _____

7. _____

   _____

8. _____

   _____

9. _____

   _____

10. _____

    _____

11. _____

    _____

12. _____

    _____

13. _____

    _____

14. _____

    _____

15. _____

    _____

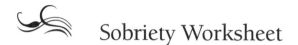

# Sobriety Worksheet

Now that you have come this far along the gentle path, it's time to create a sobriety worksheet to keep your recovery on course. This worksheet will be an exceptionally valuable tool to use as a reference guide in the weeks and months to come. Review it regularly.

Here are the basic directions with some very simple examples:

1.  Specify a list of concrete sobriety boundaries in the list provided on page 292.

    Example: No use of alcohol or other drugs.

2.  List specific behaviors that could jeopardize or endanger your ability to preserve your boundary.

    Example: Boundaries—Drinking any alcohol. Smoking pot. Danger Zones—Getting too hungry, angry, lonely, or tired. Talking to my parents about certain touchy subjects.

3.  Take each sobriety boundary and complete a sobriety worksheet for each one. Start by entering the boundary on the designated line. Record the last date of that behavior on the sobriety date line.

    Example: Drinking alcohol. February 2, 1986

4.  For each individual boundary, record the actual behaviors that would constitute a slip and require a revision of your sobriety date. Focus on those specific behaviors that were part of your addictive life. Record on the line labeled "Behaviors That Equal a Slip."

    Example: Drinking beer at my favorite bar.

5.  Next, list the behaviors that are not actual slips, but would detract from, or endanger, your sobriety. These are the behaviors that usually occurred before the actual addictive behavior. In other words, these are the things you usually did before a certain acting out or binge. Realizing this, you also know that these are potentially seductive behaviors and can lead you into a real danger zone. Record on the line labeled "Behaviors That Endanger Sobriety Boundary."

    Example: Going to my favorite bar, but not drinking beer.

6.  Fantasy is an integral part of the addictive experience. Whether excessive daydreaming, fantasizing, or actual trancelike preoccupations, these mental states are conducive to engaging in the old bad habits. Remembering that you alone know your obsessive thoughts and that only you are responsible for protecting your sobriety, list those fantasies that are unhealthy for you. Record on the line labeled "Fantasy."

    Example: Reminiscing about good times and good beer at my favorite bar.

7.  Finally, record those positive actions you now know will affirm or strengthen your sobriety boundaries. These behaviors will serve as survival action steps to help you through the difficult times that are bound to come on the path to sobriety and serenity. Don't forget to state what you will work for. Record on the line labeled "Action Step to Strengthen, Affirm Sobriety."

    Example: When I begin thinking about going to my favorite bar, I will call my sponsor. I will schedule regular activities with good friends who don't drink.

# My Personal Sobriety Boundaries

# Sobriety Worksheet

**1**

Sobriety Boundary

Sobriety Date

Behaviors That Equal a Slip

Behaviors That Endanger Sobriety

Fantasy

Action Step to Strengthen, Affirm Sobriety

**2**

Sobriety Boundary

Sobriety Date

Behaviors That Equal a Slip

Behaviors That Endanger Sobriety

Fantasy

Action Step to Strengthen, Affirm Sobriety

# Sobriety Worksheet

**3**

Sobriety Boundary

Sobriety Date

Behaviors That Equal a Slip

Behaviors That Endanger Sobriety

Fantasy

Action Step to Strengthen, Affirm Sobriety

**4**

Sobriety Boundary

Sobriety Date

Behaviors That Equal a Slip

Behaviors That Endanger Sobriety

Fantasy

Action Step to Strengthen, Affirm Sobriety

# Gifts of the Spirit

Sponsorship is only one of the ways Twelve Step work is done. One of the messages you carry in your journey is that of recovery. By your example, you will influence others, whether you intend to or not. If you have children, this is graphically clear. They rarely do what we say, but are sure to do what we do. Like snowflakes, we are all unique. We each possess our own unique combination of talents and inner strengths. We may not be aware of all of them just yet, but we are responsible for using them to the best of our ability. It is through these gifts that we can do our greatest Twelve Step work.

Becky, our office manager, is an example. Her inner strength is that she somehow makes order out of our chaos. Her talent is quilting. Her quilts are really works of art. They are also warm, cozy, and inviting. Her designs are so unique and artfully done that people receive comfort and enjoyment just by looking at them.

We all know people who allow us to feel emotions through their music; listeners who let us pour out our happiness or sadness and know how to make us feel cared for; those who have gifts of mathematical or scientific insight that help us make sense out of the unintelligible; wonderful cooks; great mechanics.... What are your gifts?

List your gifts of the spirit, your special talents and inner strengths:

(If you have trouble thinking of them, think of a time when you had great pleasure doing something. When someone said how meaningful or wonderful it was, you were surprised, maybe a little embarrassed. You had already received enjoyment for doing it and didn't expect others to enjoy it too.)

_____

_____

_____

_____

These gifts empower us. Perhaps within these gifts lies your vision, your mission. With the guidance of a Higher Consciousness, you can use them to make the dark places light.

# Beginning Again...

Some things become obvious. By the third year of recovery, most of us learn to accept that "boring is okay." One does not have to live in perpetual crisis. In the way we used to live, chaos was a way of life. Now we work to have reserves—emotional, financial, physical, and spiritual—so that when crises do occur, they do not throw us. We have the support we need.

However, it also becomes obvious that our lives are not problem free. In fact, some of the old issues re-emerge again and again. The difference is that now we have the understanding and the skills to avoid old self-destructive patterns. Most of us sooner or later say to ourselves, "I'm tired of growing," or pray to God, "No more challenges, please!" So we search for balance between the forces in our lives, for stability and the forces for change.

Preserving that balance may bring us to a point where the program ceases to nurture us and becomes dry. How to generate new energy for program efforts is the challenge. Here are concrete actions you can take to revitalize your recovery.

**Do Service Work**     For many, the ticket for making progress in recovery has been participating in the fellowship and organizational life. Service in a group or intergroup alters your perceptions and expands awareness dramatically. "Passing it on" really does make a difference.

**Participate in National Events**     Most Twelve Step fellowships organize national conferences and retreats. For many, the effort it takes to participate is rewarded many times over. For some, attendance provides watershed-like experiences in their recovery.

**Join Another Program**     Most of us qualify to participate in another fellowship. An alcoholic, for example, has codependency issues and could dramatically change his or her life by attending Al-Anon. Resistance occurs because one does not want to be a beginner again. Joining another fellowship, for many, is exactly what is needed.

**Join a Couples Fellowship**     One of the most significant developments in the recovery groups has been the emergence of couples-oriented fellowships such as Recovering Couples Anonymous or Chapter Nine. Many have reported that joining such a fellowship with a life partner enhanced recovery dramatically.

**Change Formats**     Many groups have found that changing formats can renew group life. Individuals also can shift focus. Join a "write and share" meeting or a "spirituality-focused" group.

**Explore Your Resistance**     Sometimes we resist continuing our program efforts because, if we continued to the next issue, it would be overwhelming. Sometimes the program becomes "dry" because we really do not want to deal with something. The question to ask is, What are we avoiding?

# Reflections
## on the
## Twelfth Step

Denial is the hallmark of the immature, the insecure, the self-centered, the nonaffirmed. When Faust, the man who was willing to sell his soul to the devil and condemn himself to hell, asked his visitor who he was, Mephistopheles replied, "I am the spirit who always denies!"

—Conrad Baars, M.D.
*Born Only Once*

The Twelfth Step requires that you share your path with others. The joy of your sobriety and its life-giving reality are what you have to give. Denial is how you have lost your way in the past. Reflect on the quote above and think about how the Twelfth Step can maintain reality in your life. Think, too, about the contract between the gift you offer new members and the offer of Mephistopheles.

# Getting This Far

Getting this far means you have worked very hard and have given many gifts to yourself. You have by now integrated Twelve Step principles into your core being, have changed your life dramatically, and have a rich community of friends. Let the workbook be a record of your transformation and a celebration of your courage.

There may come a time when you feel the need to revitalize your program. You may wish to complete the workbook again. People report that using these exercises at different times in their lives generated very different experiences. Feel free to repeat them. All you need is the desire, the courage, and some blank sheets of paper.

By now, you've probably realized that there is no finish line on the gentle path through the Twelve Steps. The Steps are a process—ongoing, regenerating, renewing. In recovery, as in life generally, there are always new challenges, and you will find, if you keep reaching out, plenty of friends along the way.

My congratulations! Welcome to the beginning of the rest of your journey.

Patrick J. Carnes
Del Amo Hospital
Torrance, California

# Appendix

# A Guide for Group Use

From the beginning, *The Gentle Path* was meant to be an evolving resource for Twelve Step study. Over the past three years, groups all across the country have been using the workbook in different ways, with different goals, and with different stories to tell. We have put together some of their suggestions on what worked and what didn't work for them, and we have made some changes to the book based on their comments. Here are some of the ways *The Gentle Path* was used within a group setting:

❧ It can be used as an introduction to how the Twelve Steps work. With a guide or sponsor, this book can help you understand what the Twelve Steps mean in your life.

❧ As a study guide for renewal groups, the book has helped those in recovery reach deeper levels of understanding.

❧ For those with multiple or secondary addictions, it is a tool for exploring other sides of one's addictive self.

❧ The book can be used in therapy groups or with a therapist.

❧ It can be used simply as a resource for help in presentation of a Step talk, the same way the Twelve Steps and Twelve Traditions have been used for years.

The important component of group accountability will help you continue progressing through the book. It will be the support and encouragement of other members of the group that will get you through the difficult parts and hold you accountable to yourself in your goal of study and growth.

# Study Groups

Because every group brings its own expectations and experiences, each study group is unique. Here are some suggested variations:

❧ **Post Meeting Mini-Group** This is a smaller group that chooses to meet for an hour to an hour and a half after a main Twelve Step meeting. This has two distinct advantages. First, everyone in the group has already built a trust level from knowing each other in the main Twelve Step group. Second, it minimizes the nights away from spouses and the need for baby-sitters. By meeting in a smaller group, more in-depth work time can be spent on each individual.

❧ **Write-and-Share Meeting** In this format, one person writes a part of the assigned Step. At the meeting, this person shares what he or she has written, while the others in the group write their personal reflections on what the person has shared. Each member then takes a turn sharing reflections.

❧ **Focus Group** A focus group makes a commitment to use *The Gentle Path* as a study guide. They commit a specific number of months that they plan to work on it. These groups require a sincere commitment on each member's part. To develop the trust level that is needed, the group should be closed, meaning no new members will come into the group after its formation. They operate basically as a Write-and-Share meeting. One group of four women in Michigan took only one to three pages each week, and with everyone sharing they found a connectedness in their experiences. Others' comments became catalysts to their own thoughts and feelings. A group of six men in Texas found that it worked better for them to have one person report each week on larger sections of the book. Each member was responsible for giving feedback to the person reporting. Without having to worry about what they were going to say when their turn came, they could give that person their full attention. These groups develop a deep sense of community.

❧ **All-Day Self-Help Seminars** A group may decide to use *The Gentle Path* as the format for an all-day retreat or seminar. The format may have a presentation portion, use the workbook for the "homework," and provide structured time for sharing.

# Variations

Individuals may choose to share the entire content of what they have written, or summarize their work if the group is particularly large.

It helps to bring in outside literature that pertains to the Step being worked on. One group told us that their entire group attended retreats and seminars that dealt with topics related to the Step they were working on.

Breaking bread together has always been a way of developing community. One group, determined not to get carried away, assigned a list of cold cuts, bread, condiments, chips, and refreshments and rotated who brought the ingredient for a sandwich meal every week. Another group confessed that it was comforting to have chocolate on the table when the Steps were really emotionally difficult. Some groups choose to go for coffee or lunch after meetings.

A group of young single parents pooled their money for one babysitter on Saturday mornings and brought their children with them to the church where they met. Their children had friends to play with while their parents worked the Step.

Groups with a diverse membership, or with members new to the Twelve Step program, may need greater structure in the meeting. Opening and closing rituals, like the Serenity Prayer, or readings from various meditation books, can be familiar and comforting. A "check-in" time can be allowed at the beginning of each meeting, giving everyone a chance to say, in two or three sentences, how they are feeling or what is going on with them.

Because all addicts and coaddicts have trouble with intimacy, one group chose to "practice" being open to intimacy by holding the meetings in different group members' homes, rotating the site each month.

# Time Limits

How long will the group meet? One hour or more? It helps to have the members agree on the length of the meeting and how many weeks or months each member is willing to commit. In-depth renewal groups have taken up to two-and-a-half years to complete the workbook. The group needs to reexamine its commitment from time to time, and recommit if necessary, to get the most out of the work.

The bonding that grows in *The Gentle Path* study groups is very deep, but it can delay the start of the meeting. One group allows fifteen minutes for everyone's friendly greetings and conversation before they begin the meeting.

## Leadership

The group may choose to rotate leadership each week, month, or quarter. If only one person shares her work at a meeting, she may be the designated leader that week. The leadership method will vary with each group, but in the beginning it is important to have a group consensus. It may evolve and change without verbal discussion into what feels natural for the group. However, control can be abused or abdicated, so it is important to reexamine the group consensus from time to time.

## Feedback

A group in Colorado recommended to us that groups spend some time initially hashing out agreed-upon suggestions for feedback. By doing this, the group gets to understand individual sensitivities, and it develops trust and a feeling of safety, particularly important because the First Step work requires such total exposure of one's inner secrets. The following are suggestions that this group worked out. Use them as a model only, and develop your own additional guidelines:

1. Only one person at a time speaks, uninterrupted, always.

2. Each speaker takes the floor by stating his or her name: "I'm Ann...." Although it sounds artificial, it makes it clear whose turn it is.

3. He or she has the floor until relinquishing it by saying something like "Thanks" or "That's all."

4. When the other members are sure that the speaker is finished, ask for permission to give feedback.

5. The speaker has the right to refuse or stop feedback at any time, even if he or she has previously approved it—without having to give any explanations.

6. Try to limit feedback to reflecting on what you saw or felt, rather than providing advice or analysis. Avoid intellectualizing about your personal experiences.

7. Compassion is welcome, but remember—our feelings are our feelings. We don't need to be persuaded out of them.

8. If you have a problem with something said during someone else's time, use your own time to discuss it, or wait until after the meeting.

9. Try to avoid sarcasm or other types of aggressive or negative comments during the meeting.

## Gentleness Notes

When the work gets really deep on the First Step and the Fourth and Fifth Steps, it will be tempting to think of excuses not to go to a meeting. That is when it is most important for the group to be supportive and encouraging. Connecting on the phone during the week in a buddy system helps keep everyone working together.

Build gentleness into your group process. Allow for breaks from the work and rewards for completing each Step.

# Suggested Readings

Alcoholics Anonymous World Services, Inc. *Alcoholics Anonymous,* 3rd ed. New York, 1976.

Alcoholics Anonymous World Services, Inc. *Twelve Steps and Twelve Traditions.* New York, 1978.

Anderson, Louie. *Dear Dad: Letters from an Adult Child.* New York: Penguin Group, 1989.

Anonymous. *Hope & Recovery. A Twelve Step Guide for Healing from Compulsive Sexual Behavior.* Minneapolis: CompCare Publishers, 1987.

B., Bill. *Compulsive Overeater.* Minneapolis: CompCare Publishers, 1981.

Beattie, Melody. *Beyond Codependency: And Getting Better All the Time.* Center City, MN: Hazelden, 1989.

Becker, Ernest. *The Denial of Death.* New York: The Free Press, 1973.

Black, Claudia. *Double Duty.* New York: Ballantine Books, 1990.

Bradshaw, John. *Bradshaw On: The Family. A Reveloutionary Way of Self Discovery.* Pompano Beach, FL: Health Communications, Inc. 1988.

Bradshaw, John. *Creating Love: The Next Great Stage of Growth.* New York: Bantam Books, 1992.

Campbell, Joseph. *The Hero with a Thousand Faces.* Princeton, NJ: Princeton University Press, 1976.

Carnes, Patrick. *Don't Call It Love: Recovery from Sexual Addiction.* New York: Bantam Books, 1991.

Carnes, Patrick. *Out of the Shadows: Understanding Sexual Addiction.* Minneapolis: CompCare Publishers, 1983.

Covey, Stephen R. *The Seven Habits of Highly Effective People.* New York: Simon & Schuster, 1990.

Covington, Stephanie, and Beckett, Liana. *Leaving the Enchanted Forest: The Path from Relationship Addiction to Intimacy.* San Francisco: Harper & Row Publishers, 1988.

Earle, Ralph, and Crow, Gregory. *Lonely All the Time: Recognizing, Understanding and Overcoming Sex Addiction, for Addicts and Co-Dependents.* New York: The Philip Lief Group, Inc., 1989.

Feinstein, David, and Mayo, Peg Elliott. *Rituals for Living & Dying: How We Can Turn Loss and the Fear of Death into an Affirmation of Life.* San Francisco: Harper, 1990.

Fossum, Merle A., and Mason, Marilyn, J. *Facing Shame: Families in Recovery.* New York: W.W. Norton & Company, 1986.

Geller, Anne. *Restore Your Life: A Living Plan for Sober People.* New York: Bantam Books, 1991.

Geringer Woititz, Janet. *Adult Children of Alcoholics.* Pompano Beach, FL: Health Communications, Inc., 1983.

Goleman, Daniel. *The Meditative Mind: The Varieties of Meditative Experience.* New York: Perigee Books, 1988.

Grateful Members of Emotional Health Anonymous. *The Twelve Steps for Everyone...Who Really Wants Them*, rev. ed. Minneapolis: CompCare Publishers, 1987.

Klausner, Mary Ann, and Hasselbring, Bobbie. *Aching for Love: The Sexual Drama of the Adult Child.* San Francisco: Harper & Row, Publishers, 1990.

Larsen, Earnie. *Stage II Relationships: Love Beyond Addiction.* Center City, MN: Hazelden, 1987.

Millman, Dan. *Way of the Peaceful Warrior.* Tiburon, CA: H.J. Kramer, Inc., 1984.

Nouwen, Henri, J.M. *Reaching Out.* New York: Doubleday & Company, 1975.

Peck, M. Scott. *The Road Less Traveled.* New York: Harper & Row Publishers, 1983.

Schneider, Jennifer P. *Back from Betrayal: Recovering from His Affairs.* Center City, MN: Hazelden, 1988.

Sheperd, Scott. *Survival Handbook for the Newly Recovering.* Minneapolis: CompCare Publishers, 1988.

# Twelve Step Support Group Information

The following is a partial list of Twelve Step groups.

Alcoholics Anonymous World Services, Inc.
  Box 459
  Grand Central Station
  New York, NY 10017
  (212) 686-1100

Al-Anon Family Groups
  1372 Broadway
  New York, NY 10018
  (212) 302-7240

Co-Dependents Anonymous
  P.O. Box 33577
  Phoenix, AZ 85067-3577
  (602) 277-7991

Co-Sex Addicts (Co-SA)
  Twin Cities Co-S.A.
  P.O. Box 14537
  Minneapolis, MN 55414
  (612) 537-6904

Debtors Anonymous National Organization
  P.O. Box 20322
  New York, NY 10025-9992

Gamblers Anonymous
  National Service Office
  P.O. Box 17173
  Los Angeles, CA 90017
  (213) 386-8789

Nar-Anon
  P.O. Box 2562
  Palos Verdes Peninsula, CA 90274
  (310) 547-5800

Narcotics Anonymous
  World Service Office
  P.O. Box 9999
  Van Nuys, CA 91409
  (818) 780-3951

Overeaters Anonymous
P.O. Box 92870
Los Angeles, CA
(310) 618-8835

Recovering Couples Anonymous (RCA)
P.O. Box 11872
St. Louis, MO 63105
(314) 830-2600

Sexaholics Anonymous (SA)
International Central Office
P.O. Box 300
Simi Valley, CA 93062
(818) 704-9854

P.O. Box 1542
New York, NY 10185
(212) 570-7292

Sex and Love Addicts Anonymous (SLAA)
P.O. Box 1964
Boston, MN 02105
(617) 625-7961

Sexual Addicts Anonymous (SAA)
Twin Cities Sexual Addicts Anonymous
P.O. Box 3038
Minneapolis, MN 55403
(612) 339-0217

Sexual Compulsives Anonymous (SCA)
West Coast
P.O. Box 4470
170 Sunset Blvd., #520
Los Angeles, CA 90027
(310) 859-5585

East Coast
P.O. Box 1585
Old Chelsea Station
New York, NY 10011
(212) 439-1123

# Workshops and Seminars with Dr. Patrick Carnes

Patrick Carnes often teaches weekend retreats based on *The Gentle Path*. These are powerful experiences designed in the spirit of gentleness and care that characterizes the book. They focus on using the Steps as a way to live life more effectively and to resolve issues with family and self. For information on Gentle Path Retreats, please call 1-800-532-5648.

If you wish to receive Dr. Carnes' speaking schedule on sexual dependency, trauma recovery, or family issues, please call 1-800-551-9888.

# Excerpt from
## *Out of the Shadows:*
## *Understanding Sexual Addiction*
### By Patrick Carnes, Ph.D.

There was not only the juggling act of keeping his relationships straight. Some of these women were vital to him professionally. He exploited relationships to receive cooperation. His problem was that the women would believe that he cared for them. The professional complications were extreme. One time, he was involved with a colleague and her secretary at the same time. The secretary went in to talk to her boss about this "problem" she had. Del had to face two very angry women.

His other behaviors were also problems. In porno shops, he was sexual with a number of men in the movie booths. Worse, the shops he frequented were near the capitol where he was liable to be recognized. He vowed to stop when, sitting in a meeting in the attorney general's office, a plan was described for a raid on a local porno shop—the one he had patronized two days before. But he did not stop.

Late one evening, Del pulled up next to a young woman at a stoplight. He had always had the fantasy of picking up a woman on a street. He looked at her and she smiled at him. Del became very excited. They drove side by side for several blocks. She returned his stares at each stop sign. Soon she pulled ahead of him, turned off the road, and pulled to a stop. He followed and pulled up behind her. She waved towards him and pulled out again. Del thought she wanted him to follw.

Del's mind raced ahead to where she could be leading him. She drove in the direction of a well-known local restaurant with a popular late night bar. Convinced that was where they headed, he speculated that after a drink, they might end up at her apartment. His mind filled with fantasies, he pulled up behind her when she stopped. As he was opening his door, she leaped out of her car and dashed into the building. Surprised, he looked up to see that he was not in front of the restaurant. Rather, she had stopped at the police station three blocks away.

Horrified, Del got back in his car and raced home. While driving, he was in shock at how out of touch with reality he was. She had not been encouraging him to follow her, but was in fact frightened. He, on the other hand, was so caught up in his fantasy, he failed to notice that she was parking at a police station.

He felt a flood of remorse for subjecting the woman to a frightening ordeal. Also, he was terrified that she would accuse him of attempted rape and he would be arrested. When Del arrived home at 1:30 a.m., he was so scared that he sat and prayed. At 2:00, there was a sound of a siren in the distance. He promised God that he would change. He fantasized about what it would do to his wife and kids. Truly, it was the most desperate moment of his life. Finally, he went to bed.

When he awoke in the morning, he felt tremendous relief. He knew he was not to be picked up. He went to work and put enormous energy into his job that day. At the end of the day, he felt the need of a reward. He stopped at a massage parlor.

---

Excerpt from *Out of the Shadows: Understanding Sexual Addiction,* by Patrick Carnes, Ph.D.

Also by Patrick Carnes, Ph.D.

## Contrary to Love: Helping the Sexual Addict

This is the book that inspired the PBS series and further describes and defines sexual addiction.

Trade paperback $12.95

# Don't miss:

## Hope & Recovery: A Twelve Step Guide for Healing from Compulsive Sexual Behavior, by Anonymous

A method of recovering and regaining hope for those suffering from sexual addiction and for anyone who cares about an addict.

Trade paperback  $14.95
The workbook  $9.95

Get your copies of *Out of the Shadows, Contrary to Love,* and *Hope & Recovery* at your local bookstore, by using the order form at the back of this book or calling CompCare Publishers toll free at 1-800-328-3330.

# Other Books on the Twelve Steps from CompCare Publishers

*A Day at a Time.* This best-selling daily inspirational meditation classic is an invaluable addition to twelve step recovery.

Deluxe gift edition  $10.95
Paperback edition  $6.95
Classic hardcover  $8.95

*Twelve Months of Days: Daily Inspirations for Twelve Step People and Other Seekers,* by David Rioux. This pocket-sized book of reflections, quotes, humor, and affirmations will enrich each day of recovery. $6.95

*Sober, But Stuck: Obstacles Most Often Encountered Which Keep Us from Growing in Recovery,* by Dan F. $9.95

*Twelve Steps for Everyone,* by Grateful Members of Twelve Step Fellowships. This guide will enhance your personal growth through any of the twelve step programs. $7.95

# Order Form

| Quantity | Title | Author | Cost | Total |
|---|---|---|---|---|
| | Out of the Shadows | P. Carnes, Ph.D. | $11.95 | |
| | Contrary to Love | P. Carnes, Ph.D. | $12.95 | |
| | Hope & Recovery | Anonymous | $14.95 | |
| | Hope & Recovery Workbook | Anonymous | $ 9.95 | |
| | A Day at a Time—Deluxe Gift | Anonymous | $10.95 | |
| | A Day at a Time—Paperback | Anonymous | $ 6.95 | |
| | A Day at a Time—Classic Rust | Anonymous | $ 8.95 | |
| | Twelve Months of Days | David Rioux | $ 6.95 | |
| | Sober, But Stuck | Dan F. | $ 9.95 | |
| | Twelve Steps for Everyone | Anonymous | $ 7.95 | |
| | | | Subtotal | |
| | | | Shipping & Handling | |
| | | | Sales Tax | |
| | | | Total | |

Please call us with your credit card and order toll free 1-800-328-3330 or send check or money order to CompCare Publishers. Prices subject to change without notice.

## Shipping/Handling Charges

| | |
|---|---|
| $0 – $10 | $3.50 |
| $10.01 – $25 | $4.00 |
| $25.01 — $50 | $5.00 |
| $50.01 – $75 | $7.00 |

**Send Books to:**

Name_____

Address_____

City_____State_____Zip_____

❑ Check enclosed for $_____, payable to CompCare Publishers

❑ Charge to my credit card  ❑ Visa   ❑ Mastercard   ❑ Discover

Account #_____Exp. Date _____

Signature_____Day Phone_____

## CompCare Publishers

3850 Annapolis Lane, Suite 100, Minneapolis, Minnesota 55447-5443
612/559-4800 or toll free 800-328-3330